EMQs For MRCOG Part I

Authors

P. SINHA FRCOG, MRCPI,
P.K. GUBBALA MBBS and
M. OTIFY MBBCh, M.Sc

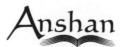
Anshan

First published in 2010 by

Anshan Ltd
11a Little Mount Sion
Tunbridge Wells
Kent. TN1 1YS

Tel: +44 (0) 1892 557767
Fax: +44 (0) 1892 530358
E-mail: info@anshan.co.uk
www.anshan.co.uk

ISBN: 978 1848290 457

British Library Cataloguing in Publication Data
A catalogue record for this book is available from the British Library

Typeset by Replika Press Pvt Ltd, India

Printed and bound in India by Replika Press Pvt. Ltd.

EMQs For MRCOG Part I

Contents

Contents

Preface

The Royal College of Obstetricians and Gynaecologists (RCOG) recently introduced Extended Matching Questions (EMQs), which have partially replaced the old style MCQs

This book contains questions with an explanation for each answer. The questions and the answers are based on the syllabus for MRCOG part 1 dictated by the RCOG.

All the questions in this book are based on scientific facts required for the part 1 exam. It is essential to practise EMQs before taking the exam. We hope this book will coach students effectively to answer EMQs.

Full details about the exam are available on the RCOG website itself.

This book follows the established format; just choose the most appropriate answer for each question. It is important to read the statements carefully to identify the theme, and select the most relevant and appropriate answer.

This book aims to cover the syllabus required to have adequate knowledge to pass the exam. We believe this book is essential for PART 1 MRCOG revision.

In the first section of the book we have written a few pages which consolidate essential knowledge on anatomy, physiology and other subjects. This is the basic knowledge necessary to answer the questions and pass the exam. In particular it is very important to remember some of the illustrated cycles and functions of the body which have been included in the book for easy revision. We have given detailed descriptions of the illustrations, for better understanding of the steps described therein.

It is advisable that you read and understand this first section of the book before embarking on the EMQ question and answer sections.

Syllabus for MRCOG Part I

The syllabus aims to cover the basic and applied sciences relevant to clinical practice based on the recommendation of the RCOG.

The topics cover a wide spectrum of anatomy, physiology, pathology and endocrinology of both male and female reproductive physiology including pregnancy, maternal-foetal oxygen transport, and placental structure and function.

Basic statistics, molecular biology, single gene and chromosome abnormalities, cellular responses in disease, benign malignant gynaecological pathology and congenital infection are also included in the syllabus.

Most of these modules are dictated by the RCOG and have been drawn from the information on the RCOG website. I would recommend you the reader to consult the website for the complete detail of the syllabus and the MRCOG Part 1 examination.

How to approach EMQs

General approach to an EMQ

✓ Read the theme title

✓ Read the introductory statement and identify the keywords (may be in **Bold**)

✓ Read the first stem and write an answer without looking at the options

✓ Find that answer in the list of options

✓ If none found re-think again

✓ Start looking at options if you do not have a clue

✓ Narrow down your choices and re-think logically

Extending matching questions (EMQs) have become widely used for MRCOG examinations. They are thought to be valuable in assessing both the level and the application of knowledge.

The EMQ paper will be similar to the MCQ paper, in that there will be a question booklet and answer sheet, which candidates will complete by filling in an answer sheet (with an HB pencil only) to be read and marked by computer.

Each question in the question booklet will consist of an option list (lettered to reflect the answer sheet), a lead-in statement (which tells you clearly what to do), and then a list of one to five questions (each numbered, again to match the answer sheet). The best way to understand this format is to look at and work through the examples we are providing.

The answer sheet area will look like this:

1	[A]	[B]	[C]	[D]	[E]	[F]	[G]	[H]	[I]	[J]	[K]	[L]	[M]	[N]	[O]
2	[A]	[B]	[C]	[D]	[E]	[F]	[G]	[H]	[I]	[J]	[K]	[L]	[M]	[N]	[O]
3	[A]	[B]	[C]	[D]	[E]	[F]	[G]	[H]	[I]	[J]	[K]	[L]	[M]	[N]	[O]
4	[A]	[B]	[C]	[D]	[E]	[F]	[G]	[H]	[I]	[J]	[K]	[L]	[M]	[N]	[O]
5	[A]	[B]	[C]	[D]	[E]	[F]	[G]	[H]	[I]	[J]	[K]	[L]	[M]	[N]	[O]

Candidates should complete the answer sheet like this:

1	[A]	[B]	[C]	■	[E]	[F]	[G]	[H]	[I]	[J]	[K]	[L]	[M]	[N]	[O]
2	[A]	[B]	[C]	[D]	[E]	[F]	[G]	■	[I]	[J]	[K]	[L]	[M]	[N]	[O]
3	[A]	■	[C]	[D]	[E]	[F]	[G]	[H]	[I]	[J]	[K]	[L]	[M]	[N]	[O]
4	[A]	[B]	[C]	■	[E]	[F]	[G]	[H]	[I]	[J]	[K]	[L]	[M]	[N]	[O]
5	[A]	[B]	[C]	[D]	[E]	[F]	[G]	[H]	[I]	[J]	[K]	■	[M]	[N]	[O]

Although the answer sheet will provide 20 possible answers, the option lists for questions may not use all of these. Most option lists will provide 10 to 14 answer options. The option lists will nearly always be in alphabetical or numerical order for ease of reference; if not, they will be in the most appropriate order for quick reference.

The most important element of the format is that you must select the **single answer that best fits**. You may feel that there are several possible answers, but you must choose only the most likely from the option list. As with the MCQ paper, if you mark two or more boxes on the same question, no mark will be awarded, even if one of the answers you choose is the correct one.

About the authors

Prabha Sinha has been a consultant obstetrician and gynaecologist at East Sussex Hospital NHS Trust since 1999. She also works as an honorary consultant in foetal medicine at St. Thomas' Hospital, London. She worked as a senior lecturer in Sheffield University's teaching hospital for two years before accepting a full time consultancy post. She is very keen and interested in teaching, training and producing teaching material useful for all grades of doctors in training.

She has published many articles in peer reviewed journals and made a large number of oral and poster presentations in various national and international conferences.

She has been an examiner for the DRCOG and for the MRCOG part 2 (Royal College for Obstetricians and Gynaecologists) for the past 4 years.

She has also taught in several MRCOG revision courses held locally and in the RCOG.

She has also written an EMQ book for MRCOG part 2, and DRCOG.

This is her sixth authored book.

Phanendra Kumar Gubbala is presently pursuing his career in obstetrics and gynaecology. During his preparation for the MRCOG he felt that there are very few books available for revision on EMQs for MRCOG part 1, and this made him take the initiative to co-write this book.

Mohamed A. Otify is a registrar in obstetrics and gynaecology. During his training for part II MRCOG he was involved in formulating clinical based questions, therefore he has contributed hugely to reviewing the questions and answers in this book.

SECTION ONE

SECTION ONE

Female Anatomy

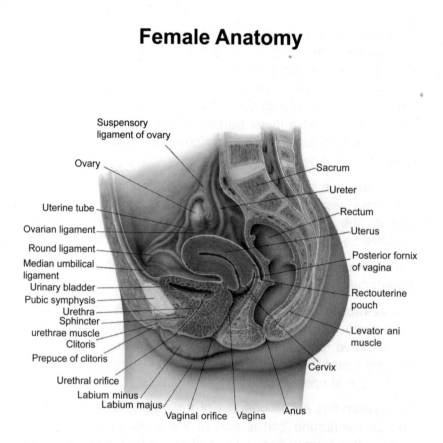

Suspensory ligament of ovary

Ovary

Uterine tube

Ovarian ligament

Round ligament

Median umbilical ligament

Urinary bladder

Pubic symphysis

Urethra

Sphincter urethrae muscle

Clitoris

Prepuce of clitoris

Urethral orifice

Labium minus

Labium majus

Vaginal orifice   Vagina   Anus

Sacrum

Ureter

Rectum

Uterus

Posterior fornix of vagina

Rectouterine pouch

Levator ani muscle

Cervix

Anatomy of external and internal female genital organs:

The female external genitalia include the structures placed about the entrance to the vagina and external to the hymen including the mons pubis (also called the mons veneris), labia majora and minora, clitoris, vestibule of the vagina, bulb of the vestibule, hymen and greater vestibular glands.

The **labia majora** are two folds of skin containing fat and loose connective tissue and sweat glands, extending from the mons pubis downward and backward to merge with the skin of the perineum. They correspond to the scrotum in the male and contain tissue resembling the dartos muscle. The round ligament connected to the uterus ends in the tissue of the labium.

The **labia minora** are also two folds of skin which are smaller and inside the labia majora on each side of the vaginal opening. In front, an upper portion of each labium minus passes over the clitoris—the structure, in the female, corresponding to the penis (excluding the urethra) in the male—to form a fold, the prepuce of the clitoris, and a lower portion passes beneath the clitoris to form its frenulum. The labia minora lack hairs but possess sebaceous and sweat glands.

The **clitoris** is a small erectile structure composed of two corpora cavernosa separated by a partition. It is partially concealed beneath the forward ends of the labia minora, possesses a sensitive tip of spongy erectile tissue, the glans clitoridis.

The external opening of the urethra is behind the clitoris and immediately in front of the vaginal opening.

The **vestibule of the vagina** is the cleft between the labia minora into which the urethra and vagina open. The **bulb** of the vestibule, corresponding to the bulb of the penis, is two elongated masses of erectile tissue that lie one on each side of the vaginal opening.

The **hymen** lies at the opening of the vagina as a thin fold of mucous membrane that is part of the vulva (external genital organs). It is formed from a layer of tissue that develops in the early stages of foetal development when the vagina is blind. This conceals the vaginal orifice and is usually incomplete (perforated with an opening). The size and shape of this opening varies greatly in each woman. An imperforate hymen can present with haematocolpos and haematometra once menstruation starts.

The hymen is usually not an indicator of virginity. The tissues are generally very thin and delicate before maturity therefore tearing of the hymen during sporting activity (bicycling, horseback riding, gymnastics) without realising it is not uncommon. Remnants of the hymen are usually present until vaginal delivery or even after.

Bartholin glands or **greater vestibular glands** are two glands located slightly below and to the left and right of the opening of the vagina. They secrete mucus to lubricate the vagina and correspond to the bulbourethral glands in the male. When a gland gets infected it results in pain and discomfort. If the duct becomes obstructed the bartholin gland becomes cystic and forms an abscess when infected. Malignant changes are extremely rare.

Development of female genital organs:

The gender of the embryo or foetus is determined by the 23rd pair of chromosomes where the egg contains X + X and the sperm contains X + Y determining the sex of the baby being a boy (foetus inherits the Y chromosome from the father) or a girl (foetus inherits the X chromosome from the father).

At six weeks the site of the genitals is a small bud, called the genital tuber. Until the ninth week the embryonic reproductive organ (internal and external genital structures) is undifferentiated and the same for the both sexes.

The embryo has two sets of organs;

1. Mullerian ducts develop into the female sex organs and

2. Wolffian ducts develop into the male sex organs

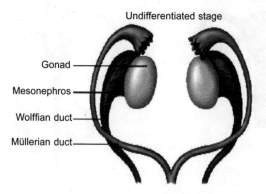

Undifferentiated stage

Gonad

Mesonephros

Wolffian duct

Müllerian duct

The development of sex organs depends on the presence of testosterone (the default sex is female). The presence of the

SRY gene, on the short arm of the Y chromosome, initiates male sexual differentiation influencing the undifferentiated gonad to form testes.

Testosterone secreted by testes stimulates the Wolffian structures (epididymis, vas deferens, and seminal vesicles), and anti-Mullerian hormone (AMH) suppresses the development of the Mullerian structures (fallopian tubes, uterus, and upper vagina).

Testosterone gets converted to dihydrotestosterone in the skin of the external genitalia which helps in masculinisation of the external genital structures.

A female embryo (XX) does not make testosterone therefore the Wolffian duct degrades, and the Mullerian duct develops into female sex organs. The clitoris is the remnants of the Wolffian duct (which develops in male sex organs).

A male embryo (XY chromosomes) which makes testosterone stimulates the Wolffian duct to develop male sex organs, and the Mullerian duct degrades. Male differentiation is mostly completed after 12 weeks. Testicles descend from the abdomen into the scrotum in the late third trimester.

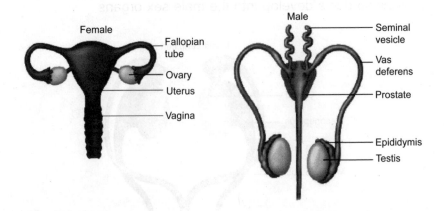

The gonads become ovaries or testicles, the phallus becomes a clitoris or a penis, and the genital folds become labia or scrotum.

In females, the gonads become ovaries; the uterus, cervix, fallopian tubes, and vagina form; the labia develop; and the phallus becomes a clitoris.

Ovaries contain over six million eggs, these decrease to approximately one million by birth and reduce to about 400 at puberty.

The Female Internal Genital Organs

The internal genital organs include the vagina, uterus, uterine tubes and ovaries.

The Vagina is a fibromuscular tube lined with stratified squamous epithelium extending from the cervix of the uterus to the vestibule of the vagina. The vagina is located posterior to the urinary bladder and anterior to the rectum and passes between the medial margins of the levator ani muscles. It pierces the urogenital diaphragm with the sphincter urethrae muscle. The posterior fibres of the sphincter urethrae muscle are attached to the vaginal wall.

Its anterior and posterior walls are normally in opposition, except at its superior end where the cervix of the uterus enters its cavity. The posterior wall is about 1 cm longer than the anterior wall and is In contact with the external os.

The cervix of the uterus projects into the superior part of the anterior wall, separating the walls of the vagina. The vaginal recess around the cervix is called the fornix (L. arch). It is divided into anterior, posterior, and lateral parts. The posterior part of the fornix is the deepest and is related to the recto-uterine or Pouch of Douglas.

The uterus lies almost at a right angle to the axis of the vagina (anteverted position). This uterine angle increases as the urinary bladder fills.

The Arterial Supply of the Vagina

The vaginal artery is usually a branch of the uterine artery. It may, however, arise from the internal iliac artery. The 2 vaginal arteries anastomose with each other and with the cervical branch of the uterine artery.

The internal pudendal artery and vaginal branches of the middle rectal artery also supply the vagina (branches of the internal iliac arteries). These arteries form anterior and posterior azygos arteries to supply the vaginal wall.

The Venous Drainage of the Vagina

The vaginal veins form vaginal venous plexuses along the sides of the vagina and within its mucosa and drains into the internal iliac veins.

They communicate with the vesical, uterine, and rectal venous plexuses.

The Lymphatic Drainage of the Vagina

The lymph vessels from the vagina are in 3 groups:

1. Those from the superior part accompany the uterine artery and drain into the internal and external iliac lymph nodes;

2. Those from the middle part accompany the vaginal artery and drain into the internal iliac lymph nodes;

3. And those from the vestibule drain into the superficial inguinal lymph nodes.

Some lymph from the vestibule drains into the sacral and common iliac lymph nodes.

Innervations of the Vagina

The vaginal nerves are derived from the uterovaginal plexus

which lies in the base of the broad ligament on each side of the supravaginal part of the cervix.

The inferior nerve fibres from this plexus supply the cervix and the superior part of the vagina which are derived from the inferior hypogastric plexus and the pelvic splanchnic nerves.

The inferior part of the vagina is supplied by the pudendal nerve.

The Uterus

This is a hollow, thick-walled, pear-shaped muscular organ (7 to 8 cm long, 5 to 7 cm wide, and 2 to 3 cm thick) located between the bladder and the rectum (in non-pregnant women). It normally projects superoanteriorly over the urinary bladder.

The wall of the uterus consists of an outer serous coat called the perimetrium. It consists of peritoneum supported by a thin layer of connective tissue; The middle muscular coat called the myometrium consists of 12 to 15 mm of smooth muscle. The myometrium increases greatly during pregnancy. The main branches of the blood vessels and nerves of the uterus are located in this layer.

The inner mucous coat called endometrium is firmly adherent to the underlying myometrium which reacts to the hormonal changes during period and sheds every month. During pregnancy, the uterus enlarges greatly to accommodate the foetus.

It consists of 2 major parts:

1. The expanded superior 2/3 is known as the body or fundus;

2. The cylindrical inferior 1/3 is called the cervix (neck of the womb).

The uterus is usually bent anteriorly (anteflexed) between the cervix and body, and it is normally bent or inclined anteriorly (anteverted). It is frequently retroverted (inclined posteriorly) in older women.

Both Fallopian tubes enter the lateral border of the body of the uterus near the fundus which is the top of the uterus. These tubes open directly into the peritoneal cavity close to the ovary.

The ligaments of the uterus include the transverse cervical ligament (cardinal ligament) extending from the cervix and lateral parts of the vaginal fornix to the lateral walls of the pelvis.

The uterosacral ligaments pass superiorly and slightly posteriorly from the sides of the cervix to the middle of the sacrum. They are deep to the peritoneum and superior to the levator ani muscles. They hold the cervix in its normal relationship to the sacrum.

The round ligaments are 10 to 12 cm long and extend for the lateral aspect of the uterus, passing anteriorly between the layers of the broad ligament. They leave the abdominal cavity through the inguinal canal and insert into the labia majora.

Broad Ligaments are a fold of peritoneum with mesothelium on its anterior and posterior surfaces extending from the sides of the uterus to the lateral walls and floor of the pelvis.

They hold the uterus in its normal position.

The broad ligament contains extraperitoneal tissue (connective tissue and smooth muscle) called parametrium and ovaries are attached through the mesovarium.

The principal support of the uterus is the pelvic floor, formed by the pelvic diaphragm. The two levator ani muscles, the two coccygeus muscles, and the muscles of the urogenital diaphragm are particularly important in supporting the uterus.

The Relationships of the Uterus

Anteriorly the body of the uterus is separated from the urinary bladder by the vesicouterine pouch where the peritoneum is reflected from the uterus onto the posterior margin of the superior surface of the bladder. The vesicouterine pouch is empty when the uterus is in its normal position.

Posteriorly the body of the uterus and the supravaginal part of the cervix are separated from the sigmoid colon by a layer of peritoneum and the peritoneal cavity. The uterus is separated from the rectum by the rectouterine pouch (of Douglas).

The inferior part of this pouch is closely related to the posterior part of the fornix of the vagina.

Laterally the relationship of the ureter to the uterine artery is very important as the ureter is crossed superiorly by the uterine artery at the side of the cervix. This is one of the important landmarks during hysterectomy.

Arterial Supply of the Uterus

This is derived mainly from the uterine arteries, which are branches of the internal iliac arteries.

They enter the broad ligaments beside the lateral parts of the fornix of the vagina, superior to the ureters.

At the isthmus of the uterus, the uterine artery divides into a large ascending branch that supplies the body of the uterus and a small descending branch that supplies the cervix and vagina. The uterine arteries pass along the sides of the uterus within the broad ligament and then turn laterally at the entrance to the uterine tubes, where they anastomose with the ovarian arteries.

The uterus is also supplied by the ovarian arteries, which are branches of the aorta.

Venous Drainage of the Uterus

The uterine veins enter the broad ligaments with the uterine arteries. They form a uterine venous plexus on each side of the cervix and its tributaries drain into the internal iliac vein. The uterine venous plexus is connected with the superior rectal vein, forming a portal-systemic anastomosis.

Lymphatic Drainage of the Uterus

The lymph vessels of the uterus follow three main routes:

1. Most lymph vessels from the fundus pass with the ovarian vessels to the aortic lymph nodes, but some lymph vessels pass to the external iliac lymph nodes or run along the round ligament of the uterus to the superficial inguinal lymph nodes.
2. Lymph vessels from the body pass through the broad ligament to the external iliac lymph nodes.
3. Lymph vessels from the cervix pass to the internal iliac and sacral lymph nodes.

Innervation of the Uterus

The nerves of the uterus arise from the inferior hypogastric plexus, largely from the anterior and intermediate part known as the uterovaginal plexus. This lies in the broad ligament on each side of the cervix.

Parasympathetic fibres are from the pelvic splanchnic nerves (S2-4), and sympathetic fibres are from the above plexus. The nerves to the cervix form a plexus in which are located small paracervical ganglia. One of these is large and is called the uterine cervical ganglion. The autonomic fibres of the uterovaginal plexus are mainly vasomotor. Most afferent fibres ascend through the inferior hypogastric plexus and enter the spinal cord via T10–12 and L1 spinal nerves.

The Fallopian Tubes are 10 cm long and 1 cm in diameter and extend laterally from the cornua of the uterus. The uterine tubes carry oocytes from the ovaries and sperm cells from the uterus to the fertilisation site in the ampulla of the tube. The tube also conveys the dividing zygote to the uterine cavity. Each tube opens at its proximal end into the cornua or horn of the uterus. At its distal end, it opens into the peritoneal cavity near the ovary and communicates between the peritoneal cavity and the exterior of the body.

The uterus is divided into 4 parts: infundibulum, ampulla, isthmus, and intramural or uterine parts.

The Infundibulum is the funnel-shaped lateral or distal end of the uterine tube closely related to the ovary and its opening into the peritoneal cavity is called the abdominal ostium. It lies at the bottom of the infundibulum which is surrounded by 20 to 30 fimbriae (L. fringes).

These finger-like processes spread over the surface of the ovary, and a large one, the ovarian fimbria, is attached to the ovary. During ovulation the fimbriae trap the oocyte and sweep it through the abdominal ostium into the ampulla.

The Ampulla begins at the medial end of the infundibulum where fertilisation of the oocyte by a sperm usually occurs. The ampulla is the widest and longest part of the uterine tube, making up over half of its length.

The Isthmus of the Fallopian Tube is the short (about 2.5 cm), narrow, thick-walled part of the uterine tube entering the cornu of the uterus.

The Intramural (Uterine) Part of the Fallopian Tube is the short segment that passes through the thick myometrium of the uterus and opens via the uterine ostium into the uterine cavity. The opening is smaller than the abdominal ostium.

The uterine tubes lie in the free edges of the broad ligaments of the uterus called mesosalpinx. Except for their uterine parts, the uterine tubes are clothed in peritoneum.

Arterial Supply of the Fallopian Tubes

The arteries to the tubes are derived from the uterine and ovarian

arteries and the branches pass to the tube between the layers
of the mesosalpinx.

Venous Drainage of the Fallopian Tubes

The veins of the tubes are arranged similarly to the arteries and
drain into the uterine and ovarian veins.

Lymphatic Drainage of the Fallopian Tubes

The lymph vessels of the uterine tubes follow those of the fundus
of the uterus and ovary and ascend with ovarian veins to the
aortic lymph nodes in the lumbar region.

Innervation of the Fallopian Tubes

The nerve supply of the uterine tubes comes partly from the
ovarian plexus of nerves and partly from the uterine plexus.
Afferent fibres from the tubes are contained in T11–12 and L1
nerves.

Embryology

Branchial arches

The first branchial arch, also called the first pharyngeal arch and the mandibular arch, is the first of six branchial arches that develops in foetal life during the fourth week of development. Is located between the stomodeum and the first pharyngeal groove?

Paired arched columns become modified into structures of the face, mandible, ear and neck.

These grow and join in the ventral midline.

The first arch, as the first to form, separates the mouth pit or stomodeum from the pericardium. By differential growth the neck elongates and new arches form, so the pharynx has six arches ultimately.

Each pharyngeal arch has a cartilaginous stick, a muscle component which differentiates from the cartilaginous tissue, an artery, and a cranial nerve. Each of these is surrounded by mesenchyme.

Arches do not develop simultaneously, but instead possess a "staggered" development.

Pharyngeal or **branchial pouches** form on the endodermal side between the arches, and **pharyngeal grooves** (or **clefts**) form from the lateral ectodermal surface of the neck region to separate the arches.

The pouches line up with the clefts; the endoderm and ectoderm remain intact and continue to be separated by a mesoderm layer.

Specific arches

There are six pharyngeal arches, but in humans the fifth arch only exists transiently during embryologic growth and development. Since no human structures result from the fifth arch, the arches in humans are I, II, III, IV, and VI.

More is known about the fate of the first arch than the remaining four. The first three contribute to structures above the larynx, while the last two contribute to the larynx and trachea.

Branchial clefts

The clefts between the branchial arches of the embryo, formed by rupture of the membrane separating corresponding endodermal pouch and ectodermal groove.

Branchial cyst

A cyst formed deep within the neck from an incompletely closed branchial cleft, usually located between the second and third branchial arches. The branchial arches develop during early embryonic life and are separated by four clefts. As the foetus develops, these arches grow to form structures within the head and neck. Two of the arches grow together and enclose the cervical sinus, a cavity in the neck. A branchial cyst may develop within the cervical sinus called also branchiogenic or branchiogenous cyst.

Branchial groove

An external furrow lined with ectoderm, occurring in the embryo between two branchial arches.

First pouch

The endoderm lines the future auditory tube, middle ear, mastoid antrum, and inner layer of the tympanic membrane.

Pharyngeal arch	Muscular contributions	Skeletal contributions	Nerve	Artery
1st (also called "mandibular arch")	muscles of mastication, anterior belly of the digastric, mylohyoid, tensor tympani, tensor veli palatini	maxilla, mandible (only as a model for mandible not actual formation of mandible), the incus and malleus of the middle ear, also Meckel's cartilage	Trigeminal nerve (V2 and V3)	Maxillary artery
2nd (also called the "hyoid arch")	Muscles of facial expression, buccinator, platysma, stapedius, stylohyoid, posterior belly of the digastric	Stapes, styloid process, hyoid (lesser horn and upper part of body), Reichert's cartilage	Facial nerve (VII)	Stapedial Artery
3rd	Stylopharyngeus	Hyoid (greater horn and lower part of body), thymus, inferior parathyroid gland	Glosso pharyngeal nerve (IX)	Common carotid/ Internal carotid
4th	cricothyroid muscle, all intrinsic muscles of soft palate except levator veli palatini	thyroid cartilage, epiglottic cartilage, superior parathyroid gland	Vagus nerve (X) Superior laryngeal nerve	Right 4th aortic arch: subclavian artery Left 4th aortic arch: aortic arch
6th	all intrinsic muscles of larynx except the cricothyroid muscle	cricoid cartilage, arytenoid cartilages, corniculate cartilage	Vagus nerve (X) Recurrent laryngeal nerve	Right 6th aortic arch: pulmonary artery Left 6th aortic arch: Pulmonary artery and ductus arteriosus

Second pouch

Contributes to the middle ear, tonsils, supplied by the facial nerve.

Third pouch

The third pouch possesses dorsal and ventral wings. Derivatives of the dorsal wings include the inferior parathyroid glands, while the ventral wings fuse to form the cytoreticular cells of the thymus. The main nerve supply to the derivatives of this pouch is cranial nerve IX, the glossopharyngeal nerve.

Fourth pouch

Derivatives include the superior parathyroid glands and parafollicular C-Cells of the thyroid gland.

Fifth pouch

Rudimentary structure becomes part of the fourth pouch contributing to thyroid C-cells.

Foetal development

Day 0	Fertilisation
Week 1	Implantation
Week 2	Bilaminar disk
Week 3	Gastrulation, primitive streak, notochord and neural plate begin to form
Week 3–8	Neural tube formed. Organogenesis
Week 4	Heart begins to beat. Limb buds begin to form
Week 10	Genitalia have male/female characteristics

Development of female genital tract

Genital tubercle (by slight elongation)	Clitoris
Genital folds (by remaining separate)	Labia minora
Genital swellings (by enlarging greatly)	Labia majora
Lower-most part of the urogenital sinus	Vestibule
Para mesonephric (mullerian) duct	Fallopian tube, uterus and part of vagina

Foetal erythropoiesis

3–8 weeks	Yolk sac
6–30 weeks	Liver
9–28 weeks	Spleen
from 28 weeks	Bone marrow

Examples of autosomal dominant conditions

Achondroplasia

Adult polycystic kidney disease

Huntington's disease

Marfan's syndrome

Familial adenomatous polyposis

Familial hypercholesterolemia

Neurofibromatosis type 1,2

Von Hippel-Lindau disease

Krebs Cycle or Tricarboxylic Acid Cycle (TCA-Cycle)

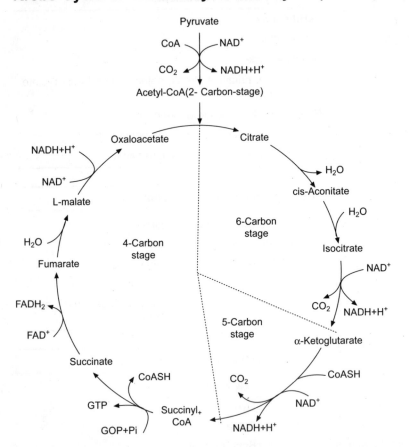

Krebs cycle: Krebs cycle (or the citric acid cycle or tricarboxylic acid cycle) is important for aerobic metabolism and involved in the breakdown of all three major groups of food (carbohydrate, fat and protein). The process occurs in mitochondria.

Glucose enters the cycle by the passage through the glycolytic pathway and conversion of acetyl CoA by the oxidative decarboxylation of pyruvate. The breakdown of glucose to carbon dioxide and water is a complex set of chemical interconversions called carbohydrate catabolism, and the Krebs cycle is the second of three major stages in the process, occurring between glycolysis and oxidative phosphorylation.

Prior to entering the Krebs cycle, pyruvate must be converted into acetyl CoA (acetyl coenzyme A). This is achieved by removing a CO_2 molecule from pyruvate and then removing an electron to reduce an NAD^+ into NADH. An enzyme called coenzyme A is combined with the remaining acetyl to make acetyl CoA which is then fed into the Krebs cycle.

The Krebs cycle is a complex series of chemical reactions in all cells that uses oxygen as part of their respiration process. The Krebs cycle produces carbon dioxide and a compound rich in energy called ATP (Adenosine triphosphate). The ATP is essential in providing cells with the energy required for the synthesis of proteins from amino acids. The pyruvate produced in glycolysis undergoes further breakdown through a process called aerobic respiration in most organisms. This process requires oxygen and yields much more energy than glycolysis.

Urea cycle

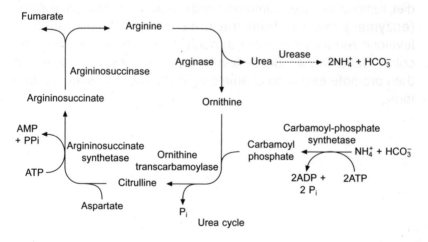

Urea cycle

The **urea cycle** (also known as the ornithine cycle) eliminates excess nitrogen from the body. In this biochemical cycle urea is formed from ammonia. The cycle primarily takes place in the liver and to a lesser extent in the kidney. In some genetic disorders (inborn errors of metabolism), and in liver failure the urea cycle is insufficient (accumulation of nitrogenous waste leading to hepatic encephalopathy). On high-protein diets the carbon skeletons of the amino acids are oxidised for energy or stored as fat and glycogen, but the amino nitrogen has to be excreted. The process is facilitated by the enzymes of the urea cycle which are controlled at the gene level. When dietary proteins increase significantly, enzyme concentration rises. On return to a balanced diet, enzyme levels decline. Under conditions of starvation, enzyme levels rise as proteins are degraded and amino acid carbon skeletons are used to provide energy. This process increases the quantity of nitrogen which should be excreted to reduce any harmful effect.

A complete lack of any one of the enzymes of the urea cycle results in death shortly after birth. However, deficiencies in each of the enzymes of the urea cycle (*N*-acetyl glutamate synthase) have been identified.

In general, the treatment requires the reduction of protein in the diet, removal of excess ammonia and replacement of intermediates (enzymes) missing from the urea cycle. Administration of levulose reduces ammonia through its action of acidifying the colon. Bacteria metabolise levulose to acidic byproducts which then promote excretion of ammonia in the faeces as ammonium ions.

Glycolysis

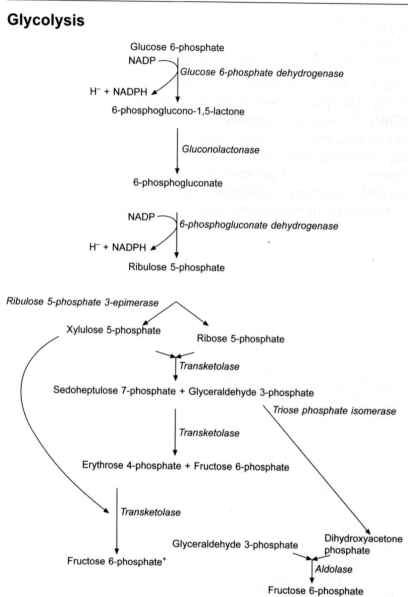

Before glucose can be converted into ATP, it has to be broken down into two pyruvate molecules (the ionized form of pyruvic acid). This process is known as glycolysis. Glycolysis takes place in the cytoplasm and can occur without the presence of oxygen. It is the primary energy source for most organisms. This process consumes two ATP molecules, and produces four ATP molecules and two $NADH_2^+$ molecules.

The first step in glycolysis is phosphorylation of glucose by a family of enzymes called hexokinases to form glucose 6-phosphate (G6P). This reaction consumes ATP, but it acts to keep the glucose concentration low, promoting continuous transport of glucose into the cell through the plasma membrane transporters. In addition, it blocks the glucose from leaking out – the cell lacks transporters for G6P. Glucose may alternatively be from the phosphorolysis or hydrolysis of intracellular starch or glycogen.

Epidemiology

- **Incidence** = Total number of new cases in a population in unit time

- **Prevalence** = incidence $\times$ disease duration

- **Sensitivity** = true positive/all people with disease

- **Specificity** = True negative/all people without disease

- **Cross-sectional study**: assesses both the health status and the exposure levels of individuals within a population at one point in time.

- **Case-control study**: a retrospective study that initially identifies two groups of subjects. All individuals in one group have the particular disease or condition under investigation (the cases), whereas everybody in the other group is free from the disease (the controls).

- **Odds ratio**: the risk of the odds of developing the disease in the exposed group divided by the odds of developing the disease in the unexposed group.

	Cases	Controls
Exposed	a	b
Not exposed	c	d

OR = (a/c)/(b/d) = ad/bc

If exposure is harmful, OR>1

If exposure is protective, OR<1

If OR = 1, no risk can be attributed to the disease

- **Cohort study**: Follows a group of subjects forward in time and compares their outcomes after one group is exposed to some known suspected cause of disease while the other group is not exposed.

- *Relative risk*: compares the risk of some health-related event occurring in two groups that are included in a prospective study. It is the probability of disease occurring in the exposed group divided by the probability of disease in the unexposed group.

	Disease present	Disease absent
Exposed	a	b
Not exposed	c	d

RR = [a/(a + b)]/[c/(c + d)]

If RR>1, association is positive

If RR<1, association is negative (or protective)

If RR = 1, not associated with risk of disease

- **Attributable risk**: the probability of disease in the exposed group minus the probability of disease in the unexposed group.

   AR = [a/(a + b)] − [c/(c + d)]

- **Absolute risk reduction**: the difference in the probability of disease between the treatment and control groups. It is calculated the same as AR, but it tells you how much of the difference in reduction of disease incidence between the groups is due to the treatment.

   ARR = [a/(a + b)] − [c/(c + d)]

- **Relative risk reduction**: the comparative reduction in rates of bad outcomes between the experimental and control groups in an RCT or cohort study.

   RRR = absolute risk reduction/probability of disease in unexposed group, thus

$$RRR = \{a/(a + b)] - [c/(c + d)]\}/[c/(c + d)]$$

- **_Number needed to treat_**: number of patients who would need to be treated in order to prevent one additional bad outcome.

$$NNT = 1/\text{Absolute risk reduction} = 1/[a/(a + b)] - (c/(c + d)]$$

Teratogenic drugs

When using drugs during pregnancy the advantages and risks of a therapy have to be considered carefully. In order to assess the risk of possible teratogenic effects the following factors have to be taken into account: the type of the drug administered, dose and duration of the medication, impaired metabolism of drugs owing to diseases of the mother, placental transfer, time of the exposure during pregnancy, genetic disposition.

High doses, administered for a short time, are extremely dangerous as they may affect the foetus. A deleterious effect on the foetus in the first trimester results in abortions and malformations, in the second and third trimester in general retardations of the foetal development, postnatal impairments of the functional development, increasing perinatal mortality, premature deliveries, stillbirths, and transplacental carcinogesis.

A long-term exposition or the administration of high doses of different substances at the end of pregnancy may produce syndromes which may possibly endanger the newborn.

Examples of some drugs and environmental chemicals which can cause teratogenic effect include:

Drugs	Effects
Alcohol	Alcohol, like other teratogens, causes a spectrum of defects. Many of the features of foetal alcohol syndrome are secondary to the effect of alcohol on brain development. These include microcephaly, short palpebral fissures, the long smooth philtrum and thin vermilion of the upper lip, joint anomalies, altered palmar crease pattern, and mental retardation.

Approximately 40% of babies born to alcoholic women and 11% of babies born to non-alcoholic but moderately drinking women have evidence of the prenatal effect of alcohol.

13-cis-retinoic acid Embryos develop reduction defects of the limb bones and an equally high percentage also have cleft palate. Limb development is most sensitive on day 11.5 of gestation while the peak susceptibility for palatal clefts begins on day 12.0. The mechanism of teratogenic action of retinoids is still far from clear.

Valproic acid Valproate is a first-line antiepileptic agent and is also used in the treatment of bipolar disorder and migraine. It is a known human teratogen. When valproate treatment cannot be avoided in the first trimester of pregnancy, the lowest effective dose should be prescribed, preferably as monotherapy, to minimize its teratogenic risk.

Neural tube defects (NTDs) are the most common of the major anomalies associated with in utero exposure to valproic acid. About 1% to 2% of exposed foetuses suffer adverse effects.

Children of women with drug treated epilepsy have lower birthweight, length, and head circumference than children of women without epilepsy.

Diethylstilbestrol Exposure to diethylstilbestrol (DES) in utero is associated with adverse effects on the reproductive tract in both male and female progeny. These effects include epididymal cysts, microphallus, cryptorchidism, testicular hypoplasia in male subjects, and adenosis, clear cell adenocarcinoma, and structural defects of the cervix, vagina, uterus, and fallopian tubes in female subjects. Strong epidemiological evidence has linked clear-cell adenocarcinoma of the vagina in young women to maternal ingestion of DES during the 1st 18 weeks of pregnancy.

Thalidomide Even a single dose of thalidomide taken during pregnancy can cause severe birth defects (physical problems present in the baby at birth) or death of the unborn baby.

Limb abnormalities are one of the most common and visible phenotypic effects of several human teratogens. The specific effects are different for most teratogens and include effects on limb morphogenesis

(e.g. thalidomide, warfarin, phenytoin, valproic acid.)

Amelia, rudimentary limb (RL), radial/tibial (RT), intercalary or central axis (CA) LD and rarely in those with terminal transverse (TT) or ulnar/fibular (UF) defects are all common with thalidomide.

Benzodiazepin   Although there are a number of studies and individual case reports concerning the use of benzodiazepines in human pregnancy, the data concerning teratogenicity and effects on postnatal development and behaviour are inconsistent.

There is evidence from studies in the 1970s that first trimester exposure to benzodiazepines in utero has resulted in the birth of some infants with facial clefts, cardiac malformations, and other multiple malformations, but no syndrome of defects.

Tumour markers

CA-125	Ovarian cancers (Epithelial tumours)
CA 19–9	Pancreatic cancers
CA 15–3	Breast cancers
CEA	Colorectal cancers, pancreatic cancer, gastric cancer
PSA	Prostate cancer
AFP	Hepatocellular cancer, non seminomatous germ cell tumour of ovary
S-100	Melanoma, neural tumours
HCG	Hydatidiform mole, choriocarcinoma and gestational trophoblastic tumours.
TRAP	(tartarate resistant acid phosphatase) hairy cell leukemia.

Tumour Suppressor Genes

BRCA 1 and BRCA 2	Breast and ovarian cancers
P 53	Li-Fraumeni syndrome and most human cancers
WT1	Wilm's tumour
APC	Colorectal cancer
Rb	Retinoblastoma
NF 1	Neurofibromatosis type 1
NF 2	Neurofibromatosis type 2

Oncogenes

bcl-2	Follicular lymphoma
c-myc	Burkitt's lymphoma
erb B2	Breast,ovarian and gastric cancer
L-myc	Lung tumour
Ret	MEN type 2 and 3
N-myc	Neuroblastoma

Stains

Ziehl-Neelsen	Acid fast bacteria
Periodic acid Schiff	Muco polysaccharides, glycogen (Whipple's Disease)
Congo red	Amyloid
Giemsa's	Borrelia, plasmodium, trypanosomes, chlamydia
India ink	Cryptococcus neoformans

Special culture mediums

Borditella pertussis	Bordet-Gengou agar
Corynebacterium diphtheria	Blood agar,Loeffler's medium,Tellurite plate
Fungi	Sabouraud's agar
Haemophilus influenza	Chocolate agar with factor V and X
Lactose fermenting enterobacterias	Pink colonies on Macconkey's agar
Legionella pneumophilia	Charcoal yeast agar buffered with iron and cystein

DNA viruses	RNA viruses
Adeno virus	Calciviruses (HEV, Norwalk virus)
Hepadnavirus (HBV)	Deltavirus (HDV)
Herpes virus (HSV1 and 2, VZV, EBV, CMV, HHV-6,7 and 8)	Flavivirus (HCV, Yellow fever, Dengue, St.Louis encephalitis, West Nile virus)
Parvovirus (B19)	Orthomyxoviruses (influenzavirus)
Papovavirus (HPV, JC)	Paramyxoviruses (Parainfluenza, RSV, Measles, Mumps)
Pox virus (small, vaccinia, molluscum contagiosum)	

Side effects of Drug

Agranulocytosis	Clozapine, carbamazepine, colchicines
Anaphylaxis	Penicillins
Aplastic anaemia	Chloramphenicol
Cardiac toxicity	Doxorubicin
Cinchonism	Quinidine, Quinine
Cutaneous flushing	Adenosine, Calcium channel blockers, Niacin, Vancomycin
Disulfiram-like reaction	Metronidazole, sulfonyl ureas and some cephalosporins
Drug induced parkinsons	Chlorpromazine, Haloperidol, Reserpine
Gynaecomastia	Cimetidine, Digitalis, Ketoconazole, Spironolactone
Haemolysis	in G6PD-deficiency (Asprin, INH, Ibuprofen, primaquine, Nitrofurantoin, Sulfonamides)
Hepatitis	INH, Halothane
Induce P-450	Barbiturates, carbamazepine, griseofulvin, phenytoin, quinidine, rifampacin
Inhibit P-450	Cimitidine, erythromycin, INH, Ketoconazole, sulfonamides
Neuro and nephrotoxicity	polymyxins
Oto and nephrotoxicity	Aminoglycosides, cisplatin, ethacrynic acid and furosemide
Pseudomembranous colitis	Clindamycin, ampicillin
Pulmonary fibrosis	Amiodarone,bleomycin and busulfan
SLE like syndrome	Hydraziline, INH, Procainamide, Phenytoin

Disease associated with neoplasm

Actinic keratosis	Squamous cell carcinoma
AIDS	Non-Hodgkin's lymphoma, Kaposi's sarcoma
Barrett's oesophagus	Oesophageal Aden carcinoma
Down's syndrome	Acute lymphoblastic leukaemia
Liver cirrhosis	Hepatocellular carcinoma
Paget's disease of bone	Osteosarcoma
Plummer-Vinson syndrome	Squamous cell carcinoma
Tuberous sclerosis	Astrocytoma and cardiac rhabdomyoma
Ulcerative colitis	Colonic adenocarcinoma
Xeroderma pigmentation	Squamous and basal cell carcinoma of skin

Antidotes

Toxin	Antidote/Treatment
Anticholinergics	Physostigmine
Benzodiazapines	Flumazenil
Paracetamol	N-acetylcysteine
Digitalis	Anti-dig Fab, Lidocaine, Mg2+, Normalize K+
Ethylene Glycol	Ethanol, Dialysis, Fomepizole
Organophosphates	Atropine, Pralidoxime
Opioids	Naloxone
Warfarin	Vit-K,FFP

Kidney hormones	Physiological function
Aldosterone	↑ Na+ reabsorption, ↑ K+ secretion, ↑ H+ secretion
Angiotensin II	↑ GFR by contracting on the efferent arteriole, ↑ Na+ and HCo3- reabsorption in proximal tubule
ANP	↓ Na+ absorption ↑ GFR
ADH	↑ water absorption in collecting ducts
Parath hormone	↑ Ca2+ absorption, ↑ phosphate reabsorption and ↓ 1,25 dihydroxy vitamin D production

Hepatitis Serology

IgM HAVb	IgM antibody to HAV(active hepatitis A)
HBsAg	Antigen for HBV, continued presence indicates carrier state
HBsAb	Antibody to HBsAg; provides immunity to hepatitis B
HBcAg	Core antigen of HBV
HBcAb	Antibody to HBcAg; positive during window period; IgM HBcAb is an indicator of recent disease
HBeAg	Antigenic determinant in HBV core; important indicator of transmissability
HBeAb	Antibody to e antigen; indicates low transmissability

Vitamin	Deficiency
Vitamin A (retinol)	Night Blindness
Vitamin B1 (thiamine)	Beri-beri, Wernicke-Korsakoff syndrome
Vitamin B2 (riboflavin)	Angular stomatitis, cheilosis
Vitamin B3 (niacin)	Pellagra
Vitamin B5 (pantothanate)	Dermatitis, enteritis, alopecia
Vitamin B6 (pyridoxine)	Convulsions and hyperirritability
Vitamin B12 (cobalamin)	Megaloblastic anaemia, optic neuropathy, sub acute combined degeneration, paresthesia
Vitamin C (ascorbic acid)	Scurvy
Vitamin D	Rickets, osteomalacia and hypocalcemic tetany
Vitamin E	Increased fragility of erythrocytes
Vitamin K	Haemorrhage
Biotin	Dermatitis, Enteritis
Folic acid	Macrocytic, megaloblastic anaemia

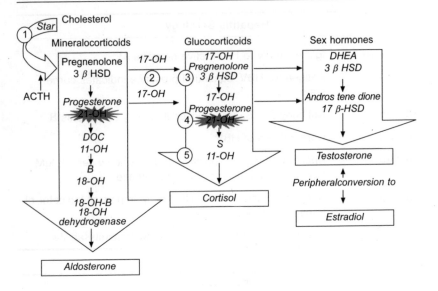

Adrenal steroidogenesis

Adrenal glands are paired situated above the kidneys and divided into cortex and medulla. The cortex is divided into three distinct zones, the outer zona glomerulosa, the middle zona fasciculata, and the inner zona reticularis. This produces three main types of hormones under the control of independent regulatory systems: glucocorticoids (cortisol), mineralocorticoids (aldosterone) and androgens (testosterone). The cortisol is synthesised in the zona fasciculata, while the mineralocorticoid aldosterone is zona glomerulosa (dependent upon enzymatic activity). Sex steroids are synthesized in the zona reticularis. Cortisol is synthesized under the trophic control of adrenocorticotropic hormone (ACTH), forming a negative feedback loop in which high serum cortisol centrally inhibits and low serum cortisol stimulates release of ACTH, which defines the hypothalamic-pituitary-adrenal axis.

Calcium metabolism

Ca is required for the proper functioning of muscle contraction, nerve conduction, hormone release, and blood coagulation. In

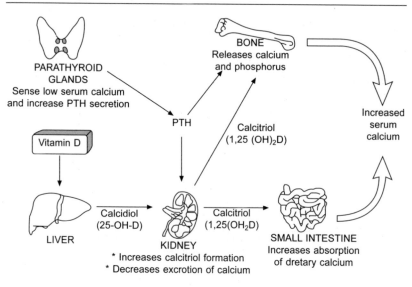

addition, proper Ca concentration is required for various other metabolic processes. Calcium metabolism is the mechanism by which the body maintains an adequate level of calcium in the blood. Derangements of this mechanism lead to hypo or hypercalcaemia which have important consequences for health.

Calcium is the most abundant mineral in the human body. The average adult body contains in total approximately 1 kg, (99% in the skeleton in the form of calcium phosphate salts). The extracellular fluid (ECF) contains approximately 22.5 mmol, of which about 9 mmol is in the serum. Approximately 500 mmol of calcium is exchanged between bone and the ECF over a period of twenty-four hours.

The regulation of both Ca and PO_4 balance is greatly influenced by concentrations of circulating parathyroid hormone, vitamin D, and, to a lesser extent, calcitonin. PTH is secreted by the parathyroid glands. It has several actions, but perhaps the most important is to defend against hypocalcaemia. Parathyroid cells sense decreases in serum Ca and, in response, release preformed PTH into the circulation. PTH increases serum Ca within minutes by increasing renal and intestinal absorption of Ca and by rapidly mobilizing Ca and PO_4 from bone (bone resorption). PTH enhances distal tubular Ca reabsorption independently of Na. PTH also decreases renal PO_4 reabsorption and thus increases renal PO_4 losses.

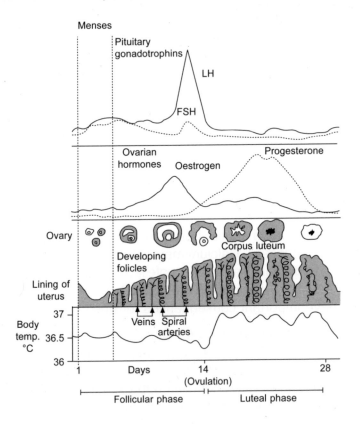

Menstrual Cycle

It is commonly divided into three phases: the follicular, mid ovulatory and luteal phase. In women, the fertile period starts at the menarche (first menstrual period) around 12 years of age and ends with the menopause, usually around 50 years. This period is divided in cycles of 28 to 35 days in length separated by menstruation. It is more by convenience than by physiological truth that the cycle starts on the first day of menstruation and ends on the day preceding the next menstruation.

The cycle is divided in two periods of unequal length: the phase that precedes ovulation (or follicular rupture) is called the follicular phase (proliferative phase) whereas the period which follows ovulation is termed the luteal phase (secretory phase). The length of the follicular phase depends on the velocity of growth of the ovarian follicles and is thus variable from one woman to another. In contrast, the length of the luteal phase depends on the lifespan of the corpus luteum, and is thus less variable. The length of each phase varies from woman to woman and cycle to cycle.

The early follicular phase starts on the first day of the cycle and ends when oestradiol begins to increase. It is characterised by increasing LH and FSH and constant low levels of oestradiol.

The late follicular phase starts with the increase in oestradiol and ends at its preovulatory peak. It is characterised by increasing oestradiol and decreasing FSH and LH levels.

The early luteal phase starts on the day of ovulation (the day after the LH peak) and ends when progesterone has reached its plateau. It is characterised by increasing progesterone and decreasing LH and FSH levels.

The mid luteal phase corresponds to *plateauing* progesterone levels. It is characterised by constant elevated progesterone and constant low levels of LH and FSH.

The late luteal phase starts when progesterone decreases and ends on the day preceding the next menses. It is characterised by decreasing progesterone and increasing LH and FSH levels. Once the oocyte has been expelled from the ruptured follicle, LH induces the secretion of progesterone from the remaining granulosa cells which organise themselves in a new gland called the corpus luteum (a process known as luteinisation). Progesterone and oestradiol increase and reach a plateau around day 22.

FSH allows recruitment and growth of the ovarian follicles as well as the selection of the dominant follicle whereas LH induces follicular rupture and sustains the corpus luteum.

An increase in oestrogen during the follicular phase stimulates the endometrium to thicken. Follicles in the ovary begin developing under the influence of a complex interplay of hormones, and after several days one or occasionally two become dominant (non-dominant follicles atrophy and die). Approximately mid-cycle, 24–36 hours after the luteinizing hormone (LH) surges, the dominant follicle ruptures and releases the ovum (ovulation). After ovulation, the egg only lives for 24 hours or less without fertilization while the remains of the dominant follicle in the ovary become a corpus luteum. This secretes progesterone which causes the endometrium to proliferate and prepare for potential implantation of a fertilized egg. If implantation does not occur within approximately two weeks, the corpus luteum involutes, causing sharp drops in levels of both progesterone and estrogen. These hormone drops cause the uterus to shed its lining in a process termed menstruation.

Infrequent or irregular ovulation is called oligoovulation. The absence of ovulation is called anovulation. Normal menstrual flow can occur without ovulation preceding it: an anovulatory cycle. In some cycles, follicular development may start but not be completed; nevertheless, oestrogen will form and will stimulate the uterine lining. Anovulatory flow resulting from a very thick endometrium caused by prolonged, continued high oestrogen levels is called oestrogen breakthrough bleeding. Anovulatory bleeding triggered by a sudden drop in oestrogen levels is called oestrogen withdrawal bleeding.

Anovulatory cycles commonly occur prior to menopause (perimenopause) and in women with polycystic ovary syndrome. Very little flow (less than 10 ml) is called hypomenorrhoea and amounts in excess of 80 ml are termed menorrhagia. Regular cycles with intervals of 21 days or fewer are called polymenorrhoea. Frequent but irregular menstruation is known as metrorrhagia.

Amenorrhoea refers to the absence of menses for more than three to six months (without pregnancy) while oligomenorrhoea is the term for cycles with intervals exceeding 35 days.

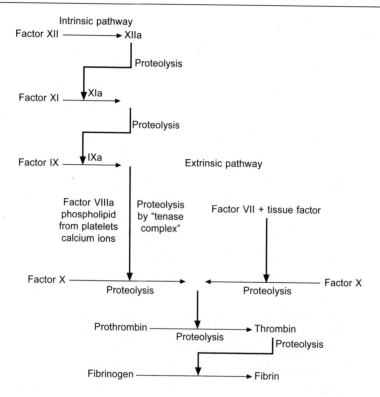

Coagulation Cascade

Coagulation (also called haemostasis) is a complex process by which blood clots. It plays an important role in stopping bleeding from a damaged vessel. Platelet and fibrin accumulates at the damaged wall of the vessel which helps in stopping the bleeding and repairs the damaged wall. Platelets immediately form a plug at the site of injury; this is called primary haemostasis followed by secondary haemostasis. Plasma protein (coagulation or clotting factor) responds in a complex cascade to form fibrin strands which strengthen the platelet plug already formed.

It begins almost instantly after an injury has caused damage to the blood vessel. The lining of the vessel (endothelium) releases phospholipid components called tissue factor and fibrinogen which initiate the chain reaction. Coagulation involves both a cellular (platelet) and a protein (coagulation factor) component.

Disorders of coagulation lead to an increased risk of bleeding or haemorrhage or clot formation. The ability of the body to control the flow of blood following vascular injury is paramount to continued survival. The process of blood clotting and then the subsequent dissolution of the clot, following repair of the injured tissue, is termed haemostasis.

It is composed of 4 major events that occur in a set order following the loss of vascular integrity:

1. The initial phase is vascular constriction which limits the blood flow of to the area of injury.

2. Platelets become activated by thrombin and aggregate at the site of injury, forming a temporary, loose platelet plug. The protein fibrinogen is primarily responsible for stimulating platelet clumping. When platelets are activated they release the nucleotide, ADP and the eicosanoid, TXA_2 (both of which activate additional platelets), serotonin, phospholipids, lipoproteins, and other proteins important for the coagulation cascade.

3. To insure stability of the initially loose platelet plug, a fibrin mesh (also called the clot) forms and entraps the plug. If the plug contains only platelets it is termed a white thrombus; if red blood cells are present it is called a red thrombus.

4. Finally, the clot must be dissolved in order for normal blood flow to resume following tissue repair. The dissolution of the clot occurs through the action of plasmin.

Damage to the blood vessel walls exposes subendothelium proteins (Von Willebrand factor), which forms a layer between the endothelium and underlying basement membrane. Von Willebrand factor recruits Factor VIII, collagen, and other clotting factors.

Circulating platelets bind to collagen with surface collagen-specific glucoprotein Ia/IIa receptors. Glycoprotein Ib/IX/V and the collagen fibril are further strengthened and these adhesions further activate the platelets.

The coagulation cascade of secondary haemostasis has two pathways, the contact activation pathway (formerly known as the intrinsic pathway), and the tissue factor pathway (formerly known as the extrinsic pathway), which lead to fibrin formation. It was previously thought that the coagulation cascade consisted of two pathways of equal importance joined to a common pathway. It is now known that the primary pathway for the initiation of blood coagulation is the tissue factor pathway. The coagulation cascade is classically divided into three pathways. The tissue factor and contact activation pathways both activate the "final common pathway" of factor X, thrombin and fibrin.

Lung Volumes

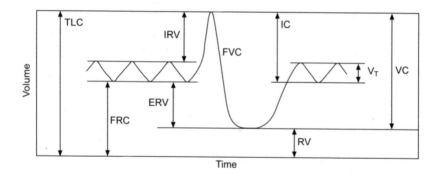

TLC – Total lung capacity, FRC – Functional residual capacity, ERV – expiratory reserve volume, IC – Inspiratory capacity, RV – Residual volume, VT – Tidal volume., FVC – Functional vital capacity

Lung volumes refer to physical differences in lung volume, while lung capacities represent different combinations of lung volumes, usually in relation to inhalation and exhalation.

The average lung can hold about 6 litres of air, but only a small amount of this capacity is used during normal breathing.

One of the most useful measurements of lung volume is vital capacity: the maximal volume of air that can be forcefully exhaled after taking the deepest breath.

TLC – Total lung capacity is the volume of air contained in the lung at the end of maximal inspiration.

FRC – Functional residual capacity is the amount of air left in the lungs after a tidal breath out and stays in the lungs during normal breathing.

ERV – Expiratory reserve volume is the amount of additional air that can be pushed out after the end expiratory level of normal breathing. (At the end of a normal breath, the lungs contain the residual volume plus the expiratory reserve volume, or around 2.4 litres. If one then goes on and exhales as much as possible, only the residual volume of 1.2 litres remains).

IC – Inspiratory capacity is the maximal volume that can be inspired following a normal expiration.

RV – Residual volume – The amount of air left in the lungs after a maximal exhalation. The amount of air that is always in the lungs and can never be expired (i.e.: the amount of air that stays in the lungs after maximum expiration)

VT – Tidal volume – The amount of air breathed in or out during normal respiration. The volume of air an individual is normally breathing in and out.

FVC – Vital capacity: The amount of air that can be forced out of the lungs after a maximal inspiration. Emphasis on completeness of expiration should be given. The maximum volume of air that can be voluntarily moved in and out of the respiratory system denotes vital capacity.

Diuretics – site of Action

Diuretics are among the most commonly used drugs. They act by diminishing sodium chloride reabsorption at different sites in the kidney (nephron), thereby increasing urinary sodium chloride

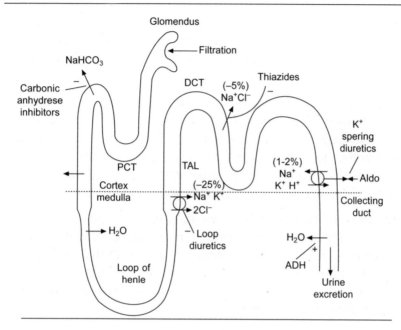

and water losses. The ability to induce negative fluid balance has made diuretics useful in the treatment of a variety of conditions, particularly oedematous states and hypertension.

The diuretics are generally divided into three major classes, which are distinguished by the site at which they impair sodium reabsorption.

Thiazide diuretics – which are the most commonly used diuretic, inhibit the sodium-chloride transporter in the distal tubule. Because this transporter normally only reabsorbs about 5% of filtered sodium, these diuretics are less efficacious than loop diuretics in producing diuresis and natriuresis.

Loop diuretics – inhibit the sodium-potassium-chloride co-transporter in the thick ascending limb. This transporter normally reabsorbs about 25% of the sodium load; therefore, inhibition of this pump can lead to a significant increase in the distal tubular concentration of sodium, reduced hypertonicity of the surrounding interstitium, and less water reabsorption in the collecting duct. This altered handling of sodium and water leads to both diuresis (increased water loss) and natriuresis (increased sodium loss). By acting on the thick ascending limb, which handles a significant fraction of sodium reabsorption, loop diuretics are very powerful diuretics.

Potassium-sparing diuretics – some drugs in this class antagonize the actions of aldosterone (aldosterone receptor antagonists) at the distal segment of the distal tubule. This causes more sodium (and water) to pass into the collecting duct and be excreted in the urine. They are called K^+-sparing diuretics because they do not produce hypokalaemia like the loop and thiazide diuretics.

Sometimes a combination of two diuretics is given because this can be significantly more effective than either compound alone (synergistic effect). The reason for this is that one nephron segment can compensate for altered sodium reabsorption at another nephron segment; therefore, blocking multiple nephron sites significantly enhances efficacy.

Foetal circulation

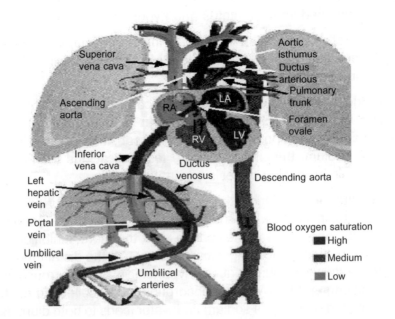

The circulation in a foetus works differently from our circulation on birth, mainly because the lungs are not in use. The foetus obtains its oxygenation and vital nutrients from the placenta via the umbilical cord. Foetal haemoglobin has a higher affinity for oxygen than adult haemoglobin, which allows a diffusion of oxygen from the mother's circulatory system to the foetus.

The foetal circulatory system is indirectly connected to the mother through the placenta, which acts as the respiratory center as well as a site of filtration for plasma nutrients and wastes from the foetus.

Blood from the placenta is carried to the foetus by the umbilical vein. About half of this enters the ductus venosus and is carried to the inferior vena cava, while the other half enters the liver. The branch of the umbilical vein that supplies the right lobe of the liver first joins with the portal vein. The blood then moves to the right atrium of the heart. In the foetus, the right and left atrium is connected by the foramen ovale. Most of the blood flows through this hole directly into the left atrium from the right atrium and bypasses the lung and continues to flow in the left ventricle. The ascending aorta circulates the blood throughout the body and also to the umbilical arteries via the internal iliac arteries. Some blood reenters the placenta where carbon dioxide and other waste products from the foetus are filtered entering the mother"s circulation. Some of the blood from the right atrium enters the right ventricle and is pumped into the pulmonary artery. In the foetus, the presence of the ductus arteriosus between the aorta and pulmonary artery directs most of this blood away from the lungs.

Derivatives of Amino acids

Arginine   −   Creatine
                     Urea
                     Nitric Oxide

Glycine   −   Porphyrin
                     Heme

Histidine   −   Histamine

Phenylalanine   −   Tyrosine
                        Thyroxine
                        Dopamine
                        Noradrenaline
                        Epinephrine
                        Melanin

Lipoproteins

Chylomicrons	Deliver triglycerides to peripheral tissues and cholesterol to liver.
LDL	Delivers hepatic cholesterol to peripheral tissues.
VLDL	Delivers hepatic triglycerides to peripheral tissues.
HDL	Reverse cholesterol transport from periphery to liver.

SECTION TWO

SECTION TWO

EMQs on Embryology

Options for questions 1–6

A	Mesonephric ducts	J	Vitelline duct
B	Paramesonephric ducts	K	Metonephron
C	Labioscrotal swelling	L	Septum transversum
D	Urogenital folds	M	Pleuro peritoneal fold
E	Genital tubercle	N	Allantois
F	Urogenital sinus	O	Ductus Venosus
G	Branchial apparatus	P	dorsal mesentry
H	Omphalo mesenteric cyst	Q	Vitelline membrane
I	Branchial arch	R	Longitudinal septum

Instruction: For each option posed below choose the single most appropriate answer from **where the organs are derived** from the A-R list above. The given option may be used once, more than once or not at all.

Question 1	Seminal vesicle
Question 2	Uterus
Question 3	Fallopian tubes
Question 4	Glans clitoris
Question 5	Labia majora
Question 6	Labia minora

Options for questions 7–12

A	Branchial arch 1	F	Branchial pouch 1
B	Branchial arch 2	G	Branchial pouch 2
C	Branchial arch 3	H	Branchial pouch 3
D	Branchial arch 4	I	Branchial pouch 4
E	Branchial cleft 1	J	Branchial pouch 5

Instruction: For each option posed below, choose the single most appropriate option from the above, **from where the organs below are derived**. Each option may be used once, more than once or not at all

Question 7	Superior parathyroid gland
Question 8	External auditory meatus
Question 9	Mandible
Question 10	Muscles of mastication
Question 11	Stapedius
Question 12	Facial nerve

Options for Questions 13–15

A	Heart begins to beat	D	Genitalia have male/female characteristics
B	Implantation of embryo	E	Fertilization by sperm
C	Organogenesis	F	Descent of testes

Instruction: For each option posed below, choose the single most appropriate option from the above **about the foetal landmarks**. Each option may be used once, more than once or not at all

Question 13	Week 10
Question 14	Week 3–8
Question 15	Week 4

EMQs on Drugs and side effects

Options for Questions: 16–19

A	Isotretinoin	J	Diethyl stilbestrol
B	Captopril	K	13-cis-retinoic acid
C	Lithium carbonate	L	Phenytoin
D	Ethanol	M	Valproic acid
E	Digoxin	N	Diazepam
F	Warfarin	O	Methimazole
G	Thalidomide	P	Tetracycline
H	Cocaine	Q	Iodide

Instruction: For the **teratogenic affects** described below, choose the single most appropriate option from the **above drugs/substances**. Each option may be used once, more than once or not at all.

Question 16	Renal damage
Question 17	Limb defects
Question 18	Vaginal clear cell carcinoma
Question 19	Dark yellow-grey teeth

EMQs on Histopathology

Options for Questions: 20–21

A	Surface ectoderm	F	Mesoderm
B	Neuroectoderm	G	Endoderm
C	Neural crest	H	Notocord

Instruction: For each option posed below, choose the single most appropriate option from the above, **from where the organs below are derived.** Each option may be used once, more than once or not at all

Question 20	Adenohypophysis
Question 21	Chromaffin cells of adrenal medulla

Options for Questions: 22–25

A	Non keratinised stratified squamous epithelium	E	Pseudostratified ciliated columnar
B	Columnar epithelium	F	Cuboidal epithelium
C	Non keratinised squamous epithelium	G	Keratinised squamous
D	Ciliated columnar epithelium	H	Transitional epithelium

Instruction: For **each organ** below, choose the single **most appropriate type of epithelium** from the above. Each option may be used once, more than once or not at all.

Question 22	Bronchus
Question 23	Ecto-cervix
Question 24	Vagina
Question 25	Fallopian tube

EMQs on Genetics and chromosomal anomaly

Options for Questions: 26–27

A	Autosomal dominant	F	X-linked dominant
B	Autosomal recessive	G	Y-linked
C	X-linked recessive	H	Mitochondrial inheritance

Instruction: For each option posed below, choose the single **most appropriate type of inheritance of the disease** from the above. Each option may be used once, more than once or not at all

Question 26	Osteogenesis imperfecta
Question 27	Glucose-6-phosphate dehydrogenase deficiency

Options for questions 28–30

A	Edward syndrome	H	Lesch-Nyhan syndrome
B	Patau syndrome	I	Gilbert's syndrome
C	Down's syndrome	J	Budd-Chiari syndrome
D	Turner's syndrome	K	Reye's syndrome
E	Hurler's syndrome	L	Klinefelter's syndrome
F	Hunter's syndrome	M	Testicular Feminisation syndrome
G	Fragile X-syndrome	N	Cri-du-chat syndrome

Instruction: For the **clinical features** described below, choose the single **most appropriate disease** from the above. Each option may be used once, more than once or not at all

Question 28	Polydactyly, cleft lip/palate, microphthalmia
Question 29	Webbed neck, coarctation of aorta
Question 30	Rocker bottom feet, low set ears, micrognathia, and clenched hand

EMQs on Epidemiology and Cancer

Options for questions 31–33

A	Smoking	G	Socio-economic status
B	HRT	H	Early menarche and late menopause
C	Oral contraceptive pills	I	Alcohol
D	Clomophine citrate	J	Cocaine abuse
E	Low fibre diet	K	Long term use of Digoxin
F	Exposure to sunlight	L	Vitamin E deficiency

Instruction: For **each gynaecological cancer** posed below, choose the single **most appropriate risk factor** from the above. Each option may be used once, more than once or not at all

Question 31	Ovarian cancer
Question 32	Endometrial cancer
Question 33	Cervical cancer

Options for questions 34–35

A	HPV 16	F	HBV
B	HPV 10	G	HAV
C	HPV 4	H	HCV
D	EBV	I	HTLV-1
E	HHV-8	J	VZV

Instruction: For each option posed below, choose the single **most appropriate virus** which is the **causative organism** from the above. Each option may be used once, more than once or not at all

Question 34	Cervical cancer
Question 35	Burkitt's lymphoma

EMQs on Infection

Options for questions 36–37

A	Primary syphilis	F	Chlamydia
B	Secondary syphilis	G	Trichomoniasis
C	Tertiary syphilis	H	Chancroid
D	Gonorrhoea	I	Condylomata acuminata
E	Genital herpes	J	Lymphogranuloma venereum

Instruction: For the **clinical features** described below, choose the single **most appropriate disease** from the above. Each option may be used once, more than once or not at all

Question 36	Painless chancre
Question 37	Painful vulvar and cervical ulcers

Options for questions 38–39

A	Antigliadin antibodies	E	Antihistone antibodies
B	Antineutrophil antibodies	F	Antibasement membrane antibodies
C	Antimicrosomal antibodies	G	Anti-epithelial cell antibodies
D	Anticentromere antibodies	H	Anti-dsDNA

Instruction: Choose the **single** most appropriate **autoantibodies** from the above **associated with the disorder** below. Each option may be used once, more than once or not at all

Question 38	SLE
Question 39	Pemphigus vulgaris

Options for questions 40–42

A	Genomic imprinting	F	Reciprocal translocation between chromosomes
B	Uniparental disomy	G	UV radiation
C	X-linked recessive	H	Mitochondrial inheritance
D	Autosomal recessive	I	Autosomal dominant
E	Multifactorial inheritance	J	Environmental factor

Instruction: For **each clinical condition** described below, choose the single **most appropriate** option from the above. Each option may be used once, more than once or not at all

Question 40	Prader-Willi syndrome
Question 41	Diabetes mellitus
Question 42	Leber's optic neuropathy

Options for questions 43–44

A	Southern blotting	F	Electrophoresis
B	Northern blotting	G	Chromatography
C	Western blotting	H	Annealing
D	Restriction endonuclease	I	South-western blotting
E	Polymerase chain reaction	J	Eastern Blotting

Instruction: For each option posed below, choose the single **most appropriate technique** from the above. Each option may be used once, more than once or not at all

Question 43	Amplification of specific DNA sequence
Question 44	DNA sequence

EMQs on Anatomy

Options for questions 45–46

A	Lateral aortic nodes	G	Sacral nodes
B	Internal iliac nodes	H	Obturator nodes
C	External iliac nodes	I	Superficial marginal nodes
D	Superficial inguinal nodes	J	Axillary nodes
E	Rectal nodes	K	Parasternal nodes
F	Deep inguinal nodes	L	Popliteal node

Instruction: For **each organ** below, choose the single **most appropriate area of lymphatic drainage** from the above. Each option may be used once, more than once or not at all

Question 45	Urethra
Question 46	Urinary bladder

Options for questions 47–50

A	T6	G	T12
B	T7	H	L1
C	T8	I	L2
D	T9	J	L3
E	T10	K	T4
F	T11	L	T5

Instruction: For each option below, choose the single **most appropriate level of openings for the passage of tubes from thorax to abdomen** from the above. Each option may be used once, more than once or not at all

Question 47	Inferior vena cava
Question 48	Oesophagus
Question 49	Aorta
Question 50	Tracheal bifurcatio

EMQs on Bacteriology

Options for questions 51–52

A	Staphylococcus spp.	H	Escherichia spp.
B	Peptostreptococcus	I	Salmonella spp.
C	Bacillus spp.	J	Pseudomonas spp.
D	Clostridium spp.	K	Bacteroides spp.
E	Neisseria spp.	L	Monobacillus spp.
F	Legionella spp.	M	Mycobacterium spp
G	Vibrio spp.	N	Chlamydia spp.

Instruction: For each option posed below, choose the single **most appropriate organism** from the above. Each option may be used once, more than once or not at all

Question 51	Gram-negative aerobic cocci
Question 52	Gram-positive anaerobic bacilli

Options for questions 53–56

A	UTI	K	Gonorrhoea
B	Meningitis	L	Syphilis
C	Opportunistic infection	M	Yaws
D	Gas gangrene	N	Q fever
E	Tetanus	O	Leptospirosis
F	Animal bites	P	Relapsing fever
G	Mesenteric adenitis	Q	Brucellosis
H	Cholera	R	Rocky mountain spotted fever
I	Plague	S	Listeriosis
J	Atypical pneumonia	T	Non-gonococcal urethritis

Instruction: For **each organism** below, choose the single **most appropriate clinical condition caused by them** from the above. Each option may be used once, more than once or not at all

Question 53	Chlamydia trachomatis
Question 54	Yersinia enterocolitica
Question 55	Coxiella burnetii
Question 56	Yersinia pestis

Options for questions 57–58

A	Yellow fever	G	Hepatitis B
B	Small pox	H	Varicella Zoster
C	Sabin polio	I	HIV
D	Measles	J	Hepatitis C
E	Mumps	K	Influenza
F	Rubella	L	Hepatitis A

Instruction: From the **clinical conditions** above, choose the single **most appropriate type of vaccine** from the below. Each option may be used once, more than once or not at all

Question 57	Killed vaccine
Question 58	Recombinant

Options for questions 59–60

A	IgG	F	IgC
B	IgA	G	IgB
C	IgM	H	IgP
D	IgE	I	IgC
E	IgD	J	IgQ

Instruction: For each option posed below, choose the single **most appropriate type of immunoglobulin** from the above. Each option may be used once, more than once or not at all

| Question 59 | Found in breast milk |
| Question 60 | Crosses the placenta |

Options for questions 61–62

A	Aflatoxins	F	Aniline dyes
B	Nitrosamines	G	Iodine
C	Asbestos	H	Alcohol
D	Arsenic	I	Polyethylene
E	Carbon tetrachloride	J	Spirit

Instruction: For **each clinical condition** described below, choose the single **most appropriate carcinogen** from the above. Each option may be used once, more than once or not at all

| Question 61 | Mesothelioma |
| Question 62 | Transitional cell carcinoma |

Options for questions 63–65

A	Cushing's syndrome	J	Scleroderma
B	Conn's syndrome	K	Tabes dorsalis
C	Addison's disease	L	Celiac sprue
D	Pheochromocytoma	M	Horner's syndrome
E	Neuroblastoma	N	Gilbert's syndrome
F	Good Pasteur's syndrome	O	Dubin-Johnson syndrome
G	Systemic lupus erythematous	P	Wilson's disease
H	Kartagener's syndrome	Q	Reye's syndrome
I	Reiter's syndrome	R	Carcinoid syndrome

Instruction: For each option posed below, choose the single **most appropriate clinical condition** from the above. Each option may be used once, more than once or not at all

Question 63	Hyponatremic volume contraction and skin hyper pigmentation
Question 64	Diarrhoea, cutaneous flushing, asthmatic wheezing.
Question 65	Calcinosis, Raynaud's phenomenon, oesophageal dysmotility, sclerodactyly and telangiectasia.

Options for questions 66–68

A	Mitochondria	F	Golgi complex
B	Ribosomes	G	Lysosomes
C	Endoplasmic reticulum	H	Phagosomes
D	Centrosome	I	Microtubules
E	Centrioles	J	Microfilaments

Instruction: For each option posed below, choose the single **most appropriate cell organelle** from the above. Each option may be used once, more than once or not at all

Question 66	Control synthesis of proteins required for intracellular metabolism
Question 67	Oxidise proteins, carbohydrates and fats in to energy.
Question 68	Facilitate intracytoplasmic transport and maintain cell shape

Options for questions 69–70

A	Epinephrine	F	Porphyrin
B	Niacin	G	Creatine
C	Serotonin	H	Urea
D	Melatonin	I	Nitric oxide
E	Histamine	J	Adrenaline

Instruction: For **each amino acid** below, choose their single **most appropriate derivative** from the above. Each option may be used once, more than once or not at all

| Question 69 | Glycine |
| Question 70 | Phenylalanine |

Options for questions 71–74

A	Vitamin B1	H	Biotin
B	Vitamin B2	I	Folate
C	Vitamin B3	J	Vitamin A
D	Vitamin B5	K	Vitamin D
E	Vitamin B6	L	Vitamin E
F	Vitamin B12	M	Vitamin K
G	Vitamin C	N	Vitamin F

Instruction: For **each clinical condition** below **caused by the deficiency of vitamins** choose the single **most appropriate option** from the above. Each option may be used once, more than once or not at all

Question 71	Wernicke-Kosakoff syndrome
Question 72	Beriberi
Question 73	Diarrhoea, dermatitis, dementia
Question 74	Macrocytic,megaloblastic anaemia

Options for questions 75–78

A	1–10 MHz	J	Cobalt-60
B	30–90 MHz	K	Cobalt-61
C	100–300 MHz	L	Cobalt-62
D	Proton	M	MRI
E	Neutron	N	Ultraviolet rays
F	Alpha particle	O	Nd-YAG laser
G	Beta particle	P	X-rays
H	Positron	Q	1 J/kg
I	Gamma ray	R	erg/g

Instruction: For each option posed below, choose the single most appropriate option from the above. Each option may be used once, more than once or not at all

Question 75	Frequencies used in diagnostic ultrasound
Question 76	Isotope associated with medicine
Question 77	Has two positive charges
Question 78	Gray (Gy.)

EMQs in Physiology

Options for questions 79–81

A	Vasopressin	F	Parathormone
B	Aldosterone	G	Vitamin D
C	Angiotensin II	H	Thyroid hormone
D	Atrial natriuretic peptide	I	Angiotensin I
E	Calcitonin	J	Renin

Instruction: For each option posed below, choose the single most appropriate option from the above. Each option may be used once, more than once or not at all

Question 79	Increases permeability to water in collecting ducts
Question 80	Increases sodium reabsorption and increases potassium secretion in distal tubule
Question 81	Decreases bone resorption of calcium.

Options for questions 82–87

A	Osteoporosis	I	Ototoxicity and nephrotoxicity
B	Extrapyramidal side effects	J	Steven-Johnson syndrome
C	Diabetes insipidus	K	SLE-like syndrome
D	Gingival hyperplasia	L	Cardiac toxicity
E	Cough	M	Fanconi's syndrome
F	Agranulocytosis	N	Cutaneous flushing
G	Gynaecomastia	O	Pulmonary fibrosis
H	Cinchonism	P	Haemolysis in G6PD-deficient patients

Instruction: For **each drug described** below, choose the single **most appropriate adverse effects caused by them** from the above. Each option may be used once, more than once or not at all

Question 82	Bleomycin
Question 83	Spironolactone
Question 84	Clozapine
Question 85	Amino glycosides
Question 86	Corticosteroids
Question 87	Lithium carbonate

Options for questions 88–91

A	GnRH	H	FSH
B	CRH	I	TSH
C	GRH	J	ACTH
D	Somatostatin	K	GH
E	TRH	L	Prolactin
F	Dopamine	M	Oxytocin
G	LH	N	Vasopressin

Instruction: For each option posed below, choose the single most appropriate option from the above. Each option may be used once, more than once or not at all

Question 88	Inhibits prolactin release
Question 89	Stimulates hepatic IGF-II synthesis and release
Question 90	Stimulates myoepithelial cells of breast causing milk let down
Question 91	Stimulates ovarian hormone synthesis and oocyte release

Options for questions 92–95

A	Rosiglitazone	G	Flutamide
B	Metformin	H	Spironolactone
C	Chlorpropamide	I	Tamoxifen
D	Goserelin	J	Clomophine citrate
E	Finasteride	K	Levonorgestrel
F	Leuprolide	L	Norgestrel

Instruction: For **each mechanism of action described** below, choose the single **most appropriate drug** from the above. Each option may be used once, more than once or not at all

Question 92	Selective oestrogen receptor modulator
Question 93	GnRH agonist
Question 94	Increase target cell response to insulin
Question 95	5-alpha reductase inhibitor

Options for questions 96–99

A	Thiamine	G	Folic acid
B	Riboflavin	H	Ascorbic acid
C	Niacin	I	Retinol
D	Pyridoxine	J	Calciferol
E	Biotin	K	Tocopherol
F	Cobalamin	L	Menaquinone

Instruction: For each option posed below, choose the single most appropriate option from the above. Each option may be used once, more than once or not at all

Question 96	Hydroxylation of collagen
Question 97	Anti-oxidant significant in fertility
Question 98	Homocysteine and methylmalonyl CoA reactions
Question 99	Formation of visual pigments

Options for questions 100–103

A	Candida albicans	G	Neisseria gonorrhoeae
B	Chlamydia trachomatis	H	Treponema pallidum
C	Herpes simplex virus	I	Trichomonas vaginalis
D	Human immunodeficiency virus	J	Pseudomonas aeruginosa
E	Gardnerella vaginalis	K	Staphylococcus aureus
F	Human papilloma virus	L	Clostridium tetani

Instruction: For **each organism described** below, choose the single most appropriate option from the above. Each option may be used once, more than once or not at all

Question 100	Non lactose fermenting, oxidase positive, gram negative rod
Question 101	Single stranded RNA virus
Question 102	Anaerobic flagellated protozoan
Question 103	Gram negative motile, spiral shaped bacterium

Options for questions 104–107

A	RSV	G	Pseudomonas aeruginosa
B	HCV	H	HBV
C	HBV	I	Legionella
D	HIV	J	HPV
E	E.coli	K	Staphylococcus saprophyticus
F	Klebsiella	L	Serratia marcescens

Instruction: For **each nosocomial infection described** below, choose the single **most appropriate causative organism** from the above. Each option may be used once, more than once or not at all

Question 104	New born nursery
Question 105	Urinary catheterisation
Question 106	Water aerosols
Question 107	Work in renal dialysis unit

Options for questions 108–110

A	PSA	F	S-100
B	CEA	G	Alkaline phosphatise
C	Alpha fetoprotein	H	Bombesin
D	HCG	I	TRAP (Tartarate resistant acid phosphatase)
E	CA-125	J	CA19–9

Instruction: For **each clinical condition** below, choose the single **most appropriate tumour marker used in the diagnosis** from the above. Each option may be used once, more than once or not at all

Question 108	Gestational trophoblastic tumours
Question 109	Hairy cell leukaemia
Question 110	Hepatocellular carcinoma

Options for questions 111–116

A	Malignant melanoma	H	Adenocarcinoma of the oesophagus
B	Thymoma	I	Squamous cell carcinoma of skin
C	Kaposi's sarcoma	J	Cardiac rhabdomyoma
D	Osteosarcoma	K	Gastric adenocarcinoma
E	Colonic carcinoma	L	Squamous and basal cell carcinoma of skin
F	Hepatocellular carcinoma	M	Acute lymphoblastic leukaemia
G	Squamous cell carcinoma of oesophagus	N	Carcinoma of the breast

Instruction: From **each clinical condition** below, choose the single **most appropriate neoplasm associated with that particular condition/disease** from the above. Each option may be used once, more than once or not at all

Question 111	Down's syndrome
Question 112	Barrett's oesophagus
Question 113	Paget's disease of bone
Question 114	Tuberous sclerosis
Question 115	AIDS
Question 116	Myasthenia gravis

Options for questions 117–121

A	Benzodiazepine	H	Protease inhibitor
B	Phenothiazine	I	Beta antagonist
C	Antifungal	J	ACE inhibitor
D	Barbiturate	K	H2-antagonist
E	Local anaesthetic	L	Alpha 1 antagonist
F	Penicillin	M	Methylxanthine
G	Tricyclic anti-depressant	N	Pituitary hormone

Instruction: For **each drug described** below, choose the single most appropriate option from the above. Each option may be used once, more than once or not at all

Question 117	Chlorpromazine
Question 118	Saquinavir
Question 119	Amitryptiline
Question 120	Theophylline
Question 121	Imipramine

Options for questions 122–125

	pH	Pco$_2$(kPa)	HCo$_3$		pH	Pco$_2$(kPa)	HCo$_3$
A	7.36	4.8	24	D	7.30	4.8	18
B	7.27	6.9	24	E	7.49	5.0	35
C	7.49	4.0	26	F	7.38	5.0	22

Instruction: For **each acid-base imbalance condition** below, choose the single most appropriate option from the above. Each option may be used once, more than once or not at all

Question 122	Metabolic acidosis
Question 123	Metabolic alkalosis
Question 124	Respiratory acidosis
Question 125	Respiratory alkalosis

Options for questions 126–128

A	Type I hypersensitivity	F	Graft versus host disease
B	Type II hypersensitivity	G	Hyper IgA syndrome
C	Type III hypersensitivity	H	Hyper IgM syndrome
D	Type IV hypersensitivity	I	Job's syndrome
E	Type V hypersensitivity	J	Chronic granulomatous disease

Instruction: For each option posed below, choose the single most appropriate option from the above. Each option may be used once, more than once or not at all

Question 126	Serum sickness
Question 127	Arthus reaction
Question 128	TB skin test

Options for questions 129–130

A	Sensitivity	F	Odds ratio
B	Specificity	G	Refinement
C	Positive predictive value	H	Suspicion
D	Negative predictive value	I	Prevalence
E	Accuracy	J	Incidence

Instruction: For **each statistical analysis described** below, choose the single **most appropriate option** from the above. Each option may be used once, more than once or not at all

Question 129	How good is this test at picking up people who have the condition?
Question 130	How good is this test at correctly excluding people without the condition?

Options for questions 131–134

A	0–10 ml	H	250–300 ml
B	20–40 ml/sec	I	400 ml
C	30–40 ml/sec	J	500 ml
D	20–30 ml	K	600 ml
E	30–40 ml	L	0–10 cm of water
F	50–60 ml	M	45–70 cm of water
G	150–200 ml	N	50–100 cm of water

Instruction: For each option posed below, choose the single most appropriate option from the above. Each option may be used once, more than once or not at all

Question 131	Residual urine
Question 132	Maximum urine flow rate
Question 133	Bladder capacity
Question 134	Voiding pressure

Options for questions 135–137

A	4 kilojoules/g	F	9 calories/g
B	6 kilojoules/g	G	4 kilocalories/g
C	9 kilojoules/g	H	6 kilocalories/g
D	4 calories/g	I	9 kilocalories/g
E	6 calories/g	J	12 kilocalories/g

Instruction: For each option posed below, choose the single most appropriate option from the above. Each option may be used once, more than once or not at all

Question 135	Carbohydrate
Question 136	Fat
Question 137	Protein

Options for questions 138–141

A	Nucleus	E	Endoplasmic reticulum
B	Nucleolus	F	Ribosomes
C	Lysosomes	G	Mitochondria
D	Golgi apparatus	H	Heterochromatin

Instruction: For **each function of a cell organelle** mentioned below, choose the single **most appropriate** option from the above. Each option may be used once, more than once or not at all.

Question 138	Contain many enzymes involved in metabolism and energy production
Question 139	Modification of proteins and their secretion and re-cycling
Question 140	Degradation of macro molecules
Question 141	Catalyse peptide bond formation in protein synthesis

Options for questions 142–145

A	HAVAb	E	HBCAb
B	HBsAg	F	HBeAg
C	HBsAb	G	HBeAb
D	HBCAg	H	HAVAg

Instruction: For each option posed below, choose the single most appropriate option from the above. Each option may be used once, more than once or not at all

Question 142	Indicator of high transmissibility
Question 143	Immunity to Hepatitis B
Question 144	Indicates low transmissibility
Question 145	Antigen associated with core of HBV

Options for questions 146–148

A	Haemophilia A	E	Bernard-Soulier disease
B	Haemophilia B	F	Glanzmann's thrombasthenia
C	Von Willebrand 's disease	G	Thrombotic thrombocytopenic purpura
D	Disseminated intravascular coagulation	H	Haemolytic uremic syndrome

Instruction: For each option posed below, choose the single most appropriate option from the above. Each option may be used once, more than once or not at all

Question 146	Factor VIII deficiency
Question 147	Factor IX deficiency
Question 148	Defect of platelet adhesion

Options for questions 149–150

A	IgG	D	IgE
B	IgA	E	IgD
C	IgM	F	IgC

Instruction: For each option posed below, choose the single most appropriate option from the above. Each option may be used once, more than once or not at all

Question 149	Found in secretions
Question 150	Crosses the placenta

Options for questions 151–153

A	Colorectal cancer	F	Li-Fraumeni syndrome
B	Osteosarcoma	G	Breast cancer
C	Wilm's tumour	H	Endometrial cancer
D	Neurofibromatosis type 1	I	Cervical cancer
E	Neurofibromatosis type 2	J	Lymphoma

Instruction: For **each tumour suppressor gene** posed below, choose the single **most appropriate associated tumour** from the above. Each option may be used once, more than once or not at all.

Question 151	Rb
Question 152	BRCA 1
Question 153	P53

Options for questions 154–156

A	N-myc	E	Ras
B	L-myc	F	Ret
C	c-myc	G	erb B2
D	bcl-2	H	D-myc

Instruction: For **each tumour**(s) described below, choose the single **most appropriate associated oncogene** from the above. Each option may be used once, more than once or not at all.

Question 154	Breast and ovarian carcinoma
Question 155	Multiple endocrine neoplasia Type II
Question 156	Burkitt's lymphoma

Options for questions 157–159

A	Charcoal yeast agar	E	Tellurite plate
B	Sabouraud's agar	F	Bordet-Gengou agar
C	Macconkey's agar	G	Thayer-Martin medium
D	Lowenstein-Jensen agar	H	Chocolate agar with factor V and X

Instruction: For **each organism** mentioned below, choose the single **most appropriate medium for isolation** from the above. Each option may be used once, more than once or not at all.

Question 157	Neisseria gonorrhoeae
Question 158	Haemophilus influenzae
Question 159	Mycobacterium tuberculosis

Options for questions 160–162

A	Acetic acid	D	Periodic acid Schiff
B	Congo red	E	India ink
C	Geimsa's	F	Ziehl-Neelsen

Instruction: Choose the single **most appropriate stains** from the above for the list option below. Each option may be used once, more than once or not at all.

Question 160	Acid-fast bacteria
Question 161	Amyloid
Question 162	Cryptococcus neoformans

Options for questions 163–164

A	Bicarbonate	E	Intrinsic factor
B	Cholecystokinin	F	Pepsin
C	Gastrin	G	Secretin
D	Gastric acid	H	Somatostatin

Instruction: For each option mentioned below, choose the single **most appropriate gastro intestinal secretory product** from the above. Each option may be used once, more than once or not at all.

| Question 163 | I cells of duodenum |
| Question 164 | Chief cells |

Options for questions 165–166

A	Proximal convoluted tubule	D	Thick descending loop of Henle
B	Distal convoluted tubule	E	Collecting tubules
C	Thin ascending loop of Henle	F	Middle convoluted tubule

Instruction: For each option posed below, choose the single most appropriate option from the above. Each option may be used once, more than once or not at all

Question 165	Reabsorbs glucose, amino acids and bicarbonate
Question 166	Reabsorbs sodium in exchange for secreting potassium or hydrogen ions

Options for questions 167–168

A	HDL	D	Chylomicron
B	LDL	E	LLD
C	VLDL	F	VHD

Instruction: For each option posed below, choose the single most appropriate option from the above. Each option may be used once, more than once or not at all

Question 167	Cholesterol transport from periphery to liver
Question 168	Delivers dietary triglycerides to peripheral tissue and dietary cholesterol to liver

Options for questions 169–171

A	Coeliac trunk	F	External iliac artery
B	Superior mesenteric artery	G	Internal iliac artery
C	Inferior mesenteric artery	H	Caecal artery
D	Abdominal aorta	I	Right colic artery
E	Common iliac artery	J	Middle colic artery

Instruction: For each option posed below, choose the single most appropriate option from the above. Each option may be used once, more than once or not at all

Question 169	Uterine artery
Question 170	Ovarian artery
Question 171	Internal pudendal artery

Options for questions 172–173

A	Stomach	H	Ovary
B	Liver	I	Anterior lobe of pituitary
C	Beta cells of pancreas	J	Posterior lobe of pituitary
D	Delta cells of pancreas	K	Hypothalamus
E	Kidney	L	Parathyroid glands
F	Adrenal glands	M	Thyroid gland
G	Colon	N	Parotid gland

Instruction: For each option posed below, choose the single most appropriate option from the above. Each option may be used once, more than once or not at all

Question 172	LH
Question 173	Oxytocin
Question 174	Insulin

Options for questions 175–177

A	Zona fasciculate	F	Liver
B	Zona glomerulosa	G	Kidney
C	Zona reticularis	H	Lung
D	Corpus luteum	I	Brain
E	Testis	J	Intestine

Instruction: For each option posed below, choose the single most appropriate option from the above. Each option may be used once, more than once or not at all

Question 175	25-hydroxylation of cholecalciferol
Question 176	Angiotensin converting enzyme is secreted
Question 177	Secretion of mineralocorticoids

Options for questions 178–180

A	Cystic fibrosis	F	Osteogenesis imperfecta
B	Down's syndrome	G	Phenylketonuria
C	Duchenne's muscular dystrophy	H	Sickle cell anaemia
D	Fragile X syndrome	I	Thalassaemia
E	Neurofibromatosis	J	Turner's syndrome

Instruction: For each **set of clinical features** described below, choose the **single most appropriate** option from the above. Each option may be used once, more than once or not at all.

Question 178	Mental retardation and large testis
Question 179	Increased susceptibility to fractures and connective tissue fragility
Question 180	Recurrent painful crisis and increased susceptibility to infections

Options for questions 181–183

A	Small cell carcinoma of lung	G	Multiple myeloma
B	Squamous cell carcinoma of lung	H	Renal cell carcinoma
C	Oligodendroglioma	I	Ependymoma
D	Breast carcinoma	J	Hemangioblastoma
E	Thymoma	K	Endometrial carcinoma
F	Lymphoma	L	Pancreatic cancer

Instruction: For each **paraneoplastic effect of tumours** below choose the single **most appropriate** option from the above. Each option may be used once, more than once or not at all

Question 181	Lambert-Eaton syndrome
Question 182	Polycythemia
Question183	Cushing's syndrome

Options for questions 184–186

A	Aplastic anaemia	F	Megaloblastic anaemia
B	Hereditary spherocytosis	G	Iron deficiency anaemia
C	Sickle cell anaemia	H	Von Willebrand's disease
D	Alpha thalassaemia	I	Bernard-Soulier disease
E	Beta thalassaemia	J	Pernicious anaemia

Instruction: For each option posed below, choose the single most appropriate option from the above. Each option may be used once, more than once or not at all

Question 184	Intrinsic factor deficiency
Question 185	Spectrin defect
Question186	Glutamic acid replaced by valine in beta-globin chain of haemoglobin

Options for questions 187–189

A	Autosomal dominant	G	Anticipation
B	Autosomal recessive	H	Pleiotropy
C	X-linked recessive	I	Variable expression
D	Mitochondrial inheritance	J	Mosaicism
E	Incomplete penetrance	K	Linkage disequilibrium
F	Anticipation	L	Dominant negative mutation

Instruction: For each option posed below, choose the **single** most appropriate option from the above. Each option may be used once, more than once or not at all

Question 187	All offspring of affected females may show signs of disease transmitted only through mother
Question 188	Age of onset of disease is earlier in succeeding generation
Question 189	No male to male transmission

Options for questions 190–192

A	Frontal lobe	G	Hypothalamus
B	Temporal lobe	H	Amygdala
C	Parietal lobe	I	Hippocampus
D	Occipital lobe	J	Midbrain
E	Cerebellum	K	Pons
F	Thalamus	L	Medulla

Instruction: For each option posed below, choose the **single** most appropriate option from the above. Each option may be used once, more than once or not at all

Question 190	Associated with visual processing
Question 191	Associated with movement, orientation, recognition, perception of stimuli
Question 192	Role in regulating states of sleep and wakefulness

Options for questions 193–194

A	Adenine	D	Cytosine
B	Guanine	E	Uracil
C	Thymine	F	Tyramine

Instruction: For each option posed below, choose the **single** most appropriate option from the above. Each option may be used once, more than once or not at all

| Question 193 | Nucleotide present only in DNA |
| Question 194 | Nucleotide present only in RNA |

Options for questions 195–196

A	M	D	G_2
B	G_1	E	G_0
C	S	F	N

Instruction: For each option posed below, choose the **single** most appropriate option from the above. Each option may be used once, more than once or not at all

Question 195	Synthesis of DNA
Question 196	Resting phase

Options for questions 197–199

A	$\alpha1$	H	D1
B	$\alpha2$	I	D2
C	$\beta1$	J	D3
D	$\beta2$	K	H1
E	M1	L	H2
F	M2	M	V1
G	M3	N	V2

Instruction: For **each physiological function** described below, choose the single **most appropriate type of receptor** from the above. Each option may be used once, more than once or not at all.

Question 197	Bronchodilatation, vasodilatation and increases glucagon release
Question 198	Increases heart rate, contractility, lipolysis and renin release
Question 199	Increases gastric acid secretion

Options for questions 200–202

	Calcium	Phosphate	Alkaline phosphatase
A	Increased	Increased	Increased
B	Normal/increased	Normal	Largely increased
C	Increased	Increased	Normal/increased
D	Normal	Normal	Normal
E	Increased	Increased	Normal

Instruction: For each option posed below, choose the single most appropriate option from the above. Each option may be used once, more than once or not at all

Question 200	Osteoporosis
Question 201	Vitamin D intoxication
Question 202	Hyperparathyroidism

Options for questions 203–207

A	Antifungal	G	H2 Agonist
B	ACE inhibitor	H	Local anaesthetic
C	Barbiturate	I	Protease inhibitor
D	Beta2 agonist	J	Penicillin
E	Benzodiazepine	K	Phenothiazine
F	Cardiac glycoside	L	Tricyclic antidepressant

Instruction: For each option posed below, choose the single most appropriate option from the above. Each option may be used once, more than once or not at all.

Question 203	Amitriptyline
Question 204	Imipramine
Question 205	Diazepam
Question 206	Phenobarbatol
Question 207	Chlorpromazine

Options for questions 208–210

A	Hypokalaemia	D	Mechanical contraction of ventricles
B	Ventricular depolarisation	E	Conduction delay through AV node
C	Ventricular repolarisation	F	Atrial depolarisation

Instruction: For each option posed below, choose the single most appropriate option from the above. Each option may be used once, more than once or not at all.

Question 208	U wave
Question 209	T wave
Question 210	P wave

Options for questions 211–214

A	Total lung capacity	E	Inspiratory reserve volume
B	Inspiratory capacity	F	Tidal volume
C	Functional reserve capacity	G	Expiratory reserve volume
D	Vital capacity	H	Residual volume

Instruction: For **each lung volume** described below, choose the single **most appropriate** option from the above. Each option may be used once, more than once or not at all

Question 211	Volume in lungs after expiration
Question 212	Air in lung at maximal expiration
Question 213	Air that moves in to lungs with each quiet inspiration
Question 214	Air that can still be breathed out after normal expiration

Options for questions 215–218

A	C3	I	L2
B	C4	J	L3
C	C5	K	L4

D	C6	L	L5
E	C7	M	S1
F	T8	N	S2
G	T9	O	S3
H	T10	P	S4

Instruction: For **each clinical reflex** below, choose the single most **appropriate nerve root** from the above. Each option may be used once, more than once or not at all.

Question 215	Patellar reflex
Question 216	Biceps reflex
Question 217	Achilles
Question 218	Triceps

Options for questions 219–220

A	C2,C3 nerve injury	E	C7 and C8 nerve injury
B	C3,C4 nerve injury	F	C8 and T1 nerve injury
C	C4 and C5 nerve injury	G	T1 and T2 nerve injury
D	C5 and C6 nerve injury	H	T2 and T3 nerve injury

Instruction: For **each nerve root injury** below, choose the single most appropriate option from the above. Each option may be used once, more than once or not at all.

Question 219	Klumpke's palsy
Question 220	Erb's palsy

Options for questions 221–223

A	Aortic stenosis	E	Ventricular septal defect
B	Aortic regurgitation	F	Patent ductus arteriosis
C	Mitral stenosis	G	Hypertrophic cardiomyopathy
D	Mitral regurgitation	H	Dilated cardiomyopathy

Instruction: For each option posed below, choose the **single** most appropriate option from the above. Each option may be used once, more than once or not at all.

Question 221	Continuous machine-like murmur
Question 222	Crescendo-decrescendo systolic ejection murmur
Question 223	Diastolic murmur with wide pulse pressure

Options for questions 224–226

A	Autosomal dominant	F	Pleiotropy
B	Autosomal recessive	G	Incomplete penetrance
C	Variable expression	H	X- Linked recessive
D	Anticipation	I	Mitochondrial inheritance
E	Imprinting	J	Dominant negative mutation

Instruction: For each option posed below, choose the **single** most appropriate option from the above. Each option may be used once, more than once or not at all.

Question 224	GOPD Deficiency
Question 225	Leber's hereditary optic neuropathy
Question 226	Huntington's chorea

EMQs based on Clinical Scenario

Options for questions 227–232

A	Neisseria gonorrhoea	J	Mycobacterium tuberclosis
B	Chlamydia trachmotis	K	Polio
C	Treponema pallidum	L	Rubella
D	Staphylococcus aureus	M	Listeria monocytogenes
E	Strept. pyogenes	N	Human papillomavirus
F	Ureaplasama	O	Calymmatobacterium granulomatis
G	Varicella zoster	P	Cytomegalovirus
H	Herpes simplex	Q	Trichomonas vaginalis
I	Rubella	R	Candida

Instructions: For **each scenario** described below, choose the **single most appropriate option from the above** list of options. Each option may be used once, more than once, or not at all.

Question 227	A 29 years old G_1 P_0 presents at 12 weeks gestation feeling unwell. She complains of fever, cough and runny nose. She discovered white spots surrounded by halo of erythema inside her mouth (buccal mucosa) as well as maculopapular rash on her abdomen.
Question 228	Two weeks old male child delivered normally (vaginal route) developed oedematous eyes, with conjunctival erythema and mucopurulent discharge.
Question 229	A 39 years old woman returned from a trip abroad where she was exposed to unprotected intercourse and more than one sexual partner for the last 3 weeks. She noticed a growth looking like a nodule over the vulva. She had no symptoms. The skin was ulcerated and appeared as a beefy red ulcer. Additional nodules had developed as well. Ulcer was painless with no enlarged lymph nodes.
Question 230	A 44 year old escort complaining of painless vulvar ulcer after having unprotected intercourse about 3 weeks ago.

| Question 231 | An infant seemingly well when he was born, showed signs of chorioretinitis, deafness, microcephaly and delayed motor milestones. |
| Question 232 | A 45 years old woman presents with inter-menstrual bleeding and menorrhagia. pipelle endometrial biopsy was performed and the pathology report suggests "Frequent giant cells, caseous necrosis and granuloma formation". |

Options for questions 233–237

A	Progesterone Implant	H	Female sterilisation
B	Vaginal ring	I	Combined contraceptive pills
C	Medroxy progesterone injectable contraception	J	Cervical cap
D	Condoms	K	Persona
E	IUCD	L	Male sterilisation
F	Natural family planning	M	Spermicides
G	LNG – Intrauterine system	N	Levonorgestrel 1.5 mg

Instructions: For **each scenario** described below, choose the **single most appropriate option from the above** list of options. Each option may be used once, more than once, or not at all.

Question 233	A 30 years old P2 who has had bad experience with the coil implant is asking for a suitable long acting reversible contraception, but she is worried about her long standing history of migraine.
Question 234	A 46 years old woman with 2 years history of menorrhagia had endometrial biopsy performed as part of the investigation, which showed simple endometrial hyperplasia.
Question 235	An 18 years old sexually active girl was tested positive for chlamydia recently. She has no stable sexual partner currently.
Question 236	A 20 years old woman presents to accident and emergency the following morning after having unprotected sexual intercourse. She is worried about getting pregnant.

Question 237	A 38 year old woman wants to have a permanent method of contraception and needs information. In addition she requires counselling regarding the failure rate of a chosen contraception method – tubal occlusion (sterilisation). She has been given the information that there is a 1 in 200 lifetime risk.

Options for questions 238–241

A	Intrauterine foetal death	F	Placenta accreta
B	Concealed haemorrhage	G	In labour
C	Abruption of placenta	H	Preterm labour
D	Antepartum haemorrhage	I	Primary postpartum haemorrhage
E	Secondary postpartum haemorrhage	J	Placenta praevia

Instructions: For **each scenario** described below, choose the **single most appropriate option from the above** list of options. Each option may be used once, more than once, or not at all.

Question 238	A 30 years old woman complains of a foul-smelling vaginal discharge 4 days after spontaneous vaginal delivery. She also gives a history of passing blood clots per vagina. On examination her BP is 90/40 mmHg, pulse 112 bpm, temperature 38.5 °C; the uterus is tender on palpation and uterine fundus above the umbilicus has moderate vaginal bleeding with blood clots ++++.
Question 239	A 29 years old pregnant woman, at 32 weeks by date, presents to the labour ward with a history of painless vaginal bleeding after intercourse. On examination: the uterus is soft and relaxed, uterus = dates; cardiotocograph (CTG) – reactive and reassuring.
Question 240	A 34 years old primigravida, who is 30 weeks pregnant, presents to the labour ward with absent foetal movements. She also complains of severe headache, epigastric pain and seeing flashes of light. On examination: BP, 170/110 mmHg; urine, protein ++++; wooden-hard uterus with no foetal movement.

Question 241	A 25 years old at 39 weeks gestation presents to the labour ward with a history of fewer foetal movements than usual during the evening. She also says that abdominal contractions are coming every few minutes and she has been having a blood stained show per vagina for the last few minutes. On vaginal examination: cervix is fully effaced, 9-cm dilated, cephalic presentation and station is +1.

Options for questions 242–245

A	Cervical swabs	F	Transabdominal ultrasound scan
B	Diagnostic hysteroscopy	G	Transvaginal USS of the pelvis, pipelle biopsy
C	Colposcopy and directed biopsy	H	Serum LH and serum FSH
D	Laparotomy	I	Pregnancy test and serum, Beta HCG
E	Hysterosalpingography	J	Diagnostic laparoscopy and dye injection

Instructions: For **each scenario** described below, choose **the single most appropriate option from the above** list of options. Each option may be used once, more than once, or not at all.

Question 242	A 60 years old post-menopausal woman, referred by GP to the gynaecological clinic with a history of irregular vaginal bleeding.
Question 243	A 28 years old woman brought by ambulance in a state of shock. Her partner informed that she had been complaining of lower abdominal pain this morning and then suddenly collapsed. He also informed that her LMP was 6–7 weeks ago. On examination her GCS score is 3, pulse 130 bpm, BP 70/35 mmHg.
Question 244	A 36 years old woman attends the gynaecological outpatient clinic with a 2-year history of primary subfertility. She also gives a history of menstrual irregularity, severe dysmenorrhoea and deep dyspareunia with normal pelvic ultrasound scan.

| Question 245 | A 44 years old woman presents to the outpatient clinic with a history of a blood stained vaginal discharge. On per speculum examination a large ulcerated mass arising from the cervix is noted. |

Options for questions 246–249

A	All children will be affected	H	All children will be carriers
B	1 in 100 will be affected	I	50% of children will be affected
C	50% of boys will be affected and 50% of girls will be carriers	J	50% of children will be carriers and 50% will be affected
D	50% of boys will be affected and all girls will be carriers	K	All girls will be affected
E	All girls will be carriers	L	All boys will be affected
F	25% of children will be affected and 25% will be normal	M	25% of children will be affected and 50% will be normal
G	25% of children will be affected and 75% will be normal	N	1 in 25 will be affected

Instructions: For **each scenario** described below, choose the **single most appropriate option from the above** list of options. Each option may be used once, more than once, or not at all.

Question 246	A 20 years old is referred to the foetal medicine unit at 13 weeks gestation. Her father has achondroplasia but she has declined genetic testing. She wants to know the risk to her unborn baby developing the disease.
Question 247	A 27 years old woman with sickle cell trait is referred to the antenatal clinic at 8 weeks gestation. Her partner is a sickle cell disease carrier. She wants to know the possible outcome.
Question 248	A 35 years old woman is referred to the antenatal clinic at 11 weeks gestation. Her father and son are affected with Haemophilia A.

| Question 249 | A 40 year old woman has a baby with Down's syndrome due to t (21:21) translocation. The woman is found to have a t (21:21) balanced translocation and is planning another pregnancy. What is the risk of having another Down's syndrome baby? |

Options for questions 250–254

A	Iron deficiency anaemia	H	Pulmonary embolism
B	Gestational diabetes mellitus	I	Impaired glucose tolerance
C	Folate deficiency	J	Thrombocytopenia
D	Bakers' cyst	K	Cholestasis of pregnancy
E	Thrombophilia	L	Acute fatty liver
F	Sickle cell disease	M	HELLP Syndrome
G	Polymorphic eruptions of pregnancy	N	Cerebrovascular stroke

Instructions: For **each scenario** described below, choose the **single most appropriate maternal condition** from the above list of options. Each option may be used once, more than once, or not at all.

Question 250	A 32 years old woman un-booked at 40 weeks delivers a 4.5kg baby by caesarean section due to failure to progress during labour. The baby needed admission to SCBU due to respiratory distress syndrome.
Question 251	A 23 years old woman presents at 35 weeks gestation with itching, pruritus mainly in palms and soles. Initial investigations show raised liver enzymes and bile acids.
Question 252	A 33 weeks pregnant patient with raised BMI of 35 presents with dyspnoea, tachypnoea, chest pain, haemoptysis and faintness.
Question 253	A 25 years old woman presented with gradual onset of headaches. Initial investigations showed raised liver enzymes, low platelets, low haemoglobin levels and ++ proteinuria. Clinical examinations reveal a tender right hypochondrium as well as lower limb oedema.
Question 254	A 28 weeks pregnant woman just had 2 hours post 75gm oral glucose load, her serum glucose concentration is found to be 12 mmol/l.

Options for questions 255–259

A	Endometrioma	G	Dermoid cyst
B	Ovarian carcinoma	H	Tubo-ovarian abscess
C	PID	I	Endometrial Ca
D	Ectopic Pregnancy	J	UTI
E	Pelvic appendix	K	Cervical cancer
F	Meigs' Syndrome	L	HELLP Syndrome

Instructions: For **each scenario** described below, choose the **single most appropriate option from the above** list of options. Each option may be used once, more than once, or not at all.

Question 255	A 34 years old woman presents with lower abdominal mass more to the left side. Ultrasound scan shows solid and cystic areas and fluid in the pouch of Douglas with evidence of pleural effusion on CT scan.
Question 256	An 18 weeks pregnant woman is found to have a mass with complex solid and cystic echo patterns during ultrasonography for lower abdominal pain.
Question 257	A lady presents with history of dysmenorrhoea and deep dyspareunia. On examination there is tenderness in the pouch of Douglas. Transvaginal scan shows cystic ovarian mass with numerous echogenic substances.
Question 258	An 18 years old, sexually active woman presents with dysuria, frequency and haematuria but no vaginal discharge.
Question 259	A 35 years old woman has been treated for pelvic inflammatory disease with IV antibiotics. After a few days she developed high temperature with dragging lower abdominal pain. Transvaginal scan shows a pelvic cystic mass.

Options for questions 260–264 ,

A	Hyperemesis gravidarum	F	Multiple pregnancy
B	Cholestasis of pregnancy	G	Pregnancy-induced hypertension
C	Acute on chronic cholecystitis	H	Intracranial tumour
D	Hydatidiform mole	I	Migraine
E	Gastroenteritis	J	Carotid artery dissection

Instructions: For **each scenario** described below, choose the **single most appropriate option from the above list** of options. Each option may be used once, more than once, or not at all.

Question 260	A G_1 P_0 patient presents at 10 weeks with vomiting, dehydration and oliguria. She does not have diarrhoea. Initial abdominal examination is unremarkable.
Question 261	A G_3 P_2 pregnant woman presents at 30 weeks with persistent headache, flashes of light as well as vomiting.
Question 262	A 28 weeks pregnant nursery carer presents with vomiting. There are reports of a few children being unwell as well.
Question 263	A 10 weeks pregnant woman presents with vomiting and vaginal bleeding admitted through the early pregnancy unit. On examination the uterus measures 16 weeks with mild tenderness as well as moderate vaginal bleeding. Transvaginal scan performed suggests enlarged uterine endometrial cavity containing innumerable anechoic cysts sized 1–30 mm.
Question 264	A 12 weeks un-booked pregnant woman presented with vomiting. On examination she was found to have a 16 weeks-sized uterus. Foetal heart sounds were present. Abdominal examination was unremarkable.

Options for questions 265–270

A	Pelvic ultrasound	**G**	Hysterosalpingogram
B	14-day course of co-amoxyclav + doxycycline	**H**	Two measurements of serum HCG 48 hours apart
C	Intrauterine device	**I**	Repeat pregnancy test
D	Laparoscopy and salpingotomy	**J**	Transfusion with type O negative blood
E	Medical management with systemic methotrexate	**K**	Immediate laparotomy
F	Endocervical swabs for culture and sensitivity	**L**	ANTI-D administered intramuscularly

Instructions: For **each scenario** described below, choose the

single most appropriate option from the above list of options.
Each option may be used once, more than once, or not at all.

Question 265	A 27 years old woman arrives in A&E by ambulance. She is unconscious with a blood pressure of 60/30 mmHg and pulse rate of 160/min. Urine is positive for beta HCG.
Question 266	A 20 years old woman attends early pregnancy unit with an 8-week history of amenorrhoea and mild vaginal bleeding. A urinary beta HCG is positive.
Question 267	A 14 weeks pregnant woman O rhesus-negative blood type presents with vaginal bleeding at 14 weeks gestation. Ultrasound scan confirms a viable pregnancy.
Question 268	A 30 years old patient with previous history of ectopic pregnancy that was treated by salpingectomy presents at 8 weeks gestation with lower abdominal pain and shoulder tip pain. Transvaginal ultrasound scan shows an empty uterus and a 2-cm diameter pulsating mass close to the right tube.
Question 269	A 33 years old woman collapses. She is extremely pale with a barely recordable blood pressure or pulse with PV bleeding.
Question 270	A 19 years old woman presents with pelvic pain 6 weeks after her last period. She had unprotected intercourse but the pregnancy test is negative. She has a mucopurulent vaginal discharge.

Options for questions 271–274

A	Spina bifida	F	Hysterosalpingogram
B	Trisomy 21	G	intra-uterine growth restriction
C	Duchene muscular dystrophy	H	Neonatal haemolysis and methaemoglobinaemia
D	Infant motor and mental developmental delay	I	Premature closure of foetal ductus arteriosus
E	Thalassaemia	J	Cerebral palsy

Instructions: For each scenario described below, choose the single most appropriate option from the above list of options. Each option may be used once, more than once, or not at all.

Question 271	A 34 years old with chronic hypertension on beta-blockers is coming for pre pregnancy counselling. She wants to know the effect of her medications on her baby.
Question 272	A 26 years old has been taking ibuprofen regularly during pregnancy for pain relief. She wants to know the effect of it on her ongoing pregnancy and on her unborn baby.
Question 273	A woman with G_1 P_0 at 12 weeks gestation takes Na-valproate to control her epilepsy. She needs to know the possible effects of that medication on her baby.
Question 274	A 27 years old woman was diagnosed with hypothyroidism at 12 weeks gestation; she refuses to take thyroxine replacement. What should she be told regarding the effect on her baby?

Options for questions 275–277

A	Detrusor instability	F	Uterine prolapse
B	Pelvic floor muscle weakness	G	Cystocoele
C	Ureterovaginal fistula	H	Rectocoele
D	Vesicovaginal fistula	I	Urethral caruncle
E	Stress urinary incontinence	J	Rectal prolapse

Instructions: For **each scenario** described below, choose the **single most appropriate option from the above** list of options. Each option may be used once, more than once, or not at all.

Question 275	A 39 years old mother of 4 children complains of incontinence when she coughs or sneezes.
Question 276	A 90 years old confused woman in a nursing home is noted by the care assistants to have spotting on the bed with a lump noted outside her vagina.
Question 277	A 43 years old with two previous normal deliveries complains of urinary frequency, nocturia and reports not being able to hold herself with sense of incomplete emptying of her bladder.
Question 278	A 55 years old had a difficult Wertheim's hysterectomy for cervical cancer. 12 weeks later she presented with unremitting urinary incontinence. This has been exacerbated during physical activities.

Options for questions 279–285

A	Perinatal mortality rate	H	Caesarean section rate
B	Stillbirth	I	Maternal survival rate
C	Coincidental maternal death	J	Indirect maternal death
D	Late maternal death	K	Maternal morbidity
E	Direct maternal death	L	Maternal near miss
F	Maternal mortality rate	M	Perinatal mortality rate
G	Early neonatal death	N	Late neonatal death

Instructions: For **each scenario** described below, choose the **single most appropriate option from the above** list of options. Each option may be used once, more than once, or not at all.

Question 279	G_1 P_0 delivered by caesarean section at 40 weeks due to abnormal CTG. She had primary post partum haemorrhage, she was transfused with 6 units of blood, 1 day later she fitted, collapsed and failed resuscitation.
Question 280	A 23 weeks pregnant woman was involved in a road traffic accident where she had a massive internal haemorrhage and died before the ambulance arrived.
Question 281	A 26 years old who is known to be hypertensive is now pregnant at 11 weeks for the first time. Her blood pressure is difficult to control. She was admitted to A&E with severe headache, blurring of vision and left-sided haemiplegia. She collapsed and failed CPR and cardioversion.
Question 282	A 39 years old delivered a male baby 2 months early. Her antenatal care was uneventful with a normal vaginal delivery and with an estimated blood loss of 300 mls. She was brought by ambulance with shortness of breath and tachycardia. She then collapsed and failed ventilation.
Question 283	A 20 years old who had a previous normal vaginal delivery comes at 25 weeks gestation with severe lower abdominal pain and vaginal bleeding. Five hours later she delivered a dead male baby.
Question 284	A 29 years old delivered had an elective Caesarean section at 39 weeks, after two previous 2 caesarean sections. She was discharged 3 days later. She slept for 5 hours at home and when she got up her baby was in his cot with no signs of life.

| Question 285 | A 21 years old had caesarean section at 41 weeks due to failed induction. The baby was admitted to special care baby unit for a systolic murmur. Then baby's condition deteriorated and required ventilation. Baby remained in SCBU for 2 weeks then died suddenly. |

Options for questions 286–292

A	Polycystic ovary syndrome	H	Edwards syndrome.
B	Kawasaki disease	I	Androgen insensitivity syndrome (AIS)
C	Arnold chiari malformation	J	Turner syndrome
D	Dandy-Walker syndrome	K	Anencephaly
E	Kleinfelter's syndrome	L	Congenital adrenal hyperplasia
F	Exomphalus	M	Down's syndrome
G	Gastroschisis	N	Patau's syndrome

Instructions: For **each scenario** described below, choose the **single most appropriate option from the above** list of options. Each option may be used once, more than once, or not at all.

Question 286	A 39 years old had amniocentesis for increased risk of Down's syndrome on nuchal translucency scan at 12 weeks. The results of the amniocentesis came back as trisomy 18.
Question 287	On a 20 weeks anomalies scan, the sonographer reported that the baby has an abnormality in the anterior abdominal wall, to the right of the umbilicus with no covering amnion. She had previously had an amniocentesis which did not show any genetic abnormality.
Question 288	A couple presents to you with history of primary subfertility for 3 years. All the female investigations look normal. Semen analysis shows azoospermia. He reports being diagnosed with gynaecomastia at the age of 14; he also reports a low sex drive. Clinical examination reveals small testis.
Question 289	A 28 years old delivers her first baby, the midwife is confused about the sex of the baby and describes it as having ambiguous genitalia.

Question 290	A 30 years old is having an anomaly scan for her second pregnancy. The baby was reported to have no skull bones as well as absent forebrain.
Question 291	A 29 years old attends infertility clinic with a history of 3 years primary sub-fertility. Initial examination shows short stature, short webbed neck, down slanting and wide epicanthic folds.
Question 292	A 24-year-old female is investigated for primary amenorrhoea. Physical examination revealed a female with normal external genitalia with the absence of uterus and cervix. The blind vagina was 3 cm long. Digital rectal examination revealed a large firm mass in the mid-pelvis.

Options for questions 293–298

A	Human papilloma virus	H	Human leucocytic virus
B	Herpes simplex virus	I	HIV
C	Rubella Virus	J	Treponame pallidum
D	H1N1 virus	K	Listeria monocytogens
E	Varicella zoster virus	L	Cytomegalovirus
F	Group B Streptococcus	M	Toxoplasmosis
G	Staphylococcus aureus	N	H. Influenza

Instructions: For **each scenario** described below, choose the **single most appropriate option from the above** list of options. Each option may be used once, more than once, or not at all.

Question 293	A $G_1 P_0$ who is at 40 weeks developed a "flu-like" illness with fever and general malaise, her baby was born with hepato-splenomegaly and jaundice.
Question 294	A woman has a history of 3 previous stillbirths, is now pregnant and at 35 weeks complains of fever and rash. Her son was born healthy but at 11 months he had abnormal incisors and later developed deafness.
Question 295	A 36 weeks pregnant patient presents with decreased foetal movement for 48 hours. An ultrasound scan confirms intrauterine foetal death. Four weeks earlier she had fever, muscle pain, joint pain, headache, stiff neck, backache, chills and sore throat for which she received ampicillin antibiotics.

Question 296	A 27 years old delivered a baby at term; the baby showed signs of distress at delivery with meconium stained liquid as well as low apgars. Early assessment showed that the baby was grunting, tachypnoeic and cyanotic with temperature instability. The paediatrician started broad spectrum antibiotics for the baby after sending cultures.
Question 297	A G_1 P_0 who is at 40 weeks develops a "flu-like" illness with fever and general malaise. She is a smoker and has got cough with dyspnoea and tachypnoea. She remembers she had a rash in the first trimester. The baby is born with microphthalmia, cataracts, limb hypoplasia, microcephaly.
Question 298	A 23 years old had a normal vaginal delivery. Three years later the baby was checked by the ENT physician who reported a lump on his vocal cord.

Options for questions 299–300

A	Sensitivity	H	Mean
B	A 95 % confidence interval	I	A 0 % confidence interval
C	Specificity	J	Multiples of the median
D	False negative	K	Null hypothesis
E	False positive	L	Paired t-Test
F	Negative predictive value	M	Probability
G	Positive predictive value	N	Chi squared test

Instructions: For **each scenario** described below, choose the **single most appropriate option from the above** list of options. Each option may be used once, more than once, or not at all.

Question 299	If zero difference lies within the 95% when comparing two groups to a treatment, it indicates the treatment has no effect.
Question 300	Out of 100,000 pregnant women, 1000 were screening positive. Of these 3 have got a Down's syndrome baby.

Section Three

Answers

Answer 1 – (A) – Seminal vesicle

Seminal vesicles develop from mesonephric or Wolffian ducts. These ducts in the embryo drain the mesonephric tubule and develop into the male sex organs.

Answer 2 – (B) – Paramesonephric duct

The uterus develops from the Mullerian or paramesonephric ducts which are a pair of embryonic ducts which become the Fallopian tubes, uterus and upper third of the vagina. Mullerian ducts develop into the female sex organs.

Answer 3 – (B) – See above

Answer 4 – (E) – Genital Tubercle

The genital tubercle develops around week 4 after fertilisation and by week 9 becomes the clitoris in the female and the penis in the male.

Answer 5 – (C) – Labioscrotal swelling

These are the paired swellings lying on each side of the developing genital tubercle and urogenital orifice prior to sex differentiation. This forms the labia majora in the female and scrotum in the male.

The labia majora are two folds of skin containing fat and loose connective tissue and sweat glands, extending from the mons pubis downward and backward to merge with the skin of the perineum. They correspond to the scrotum in the male and contain tissue resembling the dartos muscle. The round ligament connected to the uterus ends in the tissue of the labium.

Answer 6 – (D) – Urogenital fold

The labia minora in the female and ventral shaft of penis in the male develop from the urogenital fold. The labia minora are two folds of skin which are smaller and inside the labia majora lying on each side of the vaginal opening. In front, an upper portion of each labium minus passes over the clitoris - the structure in the female corresponding to the penis (excluding the urethra) in the male - to form a fold, the prepuce of the clitoris, and a lower portion passes beneath the clitoris to form its frenulum.

The labia minora lack hairs but possess sebaceous and sweat glands.

Answer 7 – (I) – Branchial Pouch 4

Superior parathyroid gland is the only structure that develops from branchial pouch 4.

There are 4 branchial pouches :-

First pouch

The endoderm lines the future auditory tube, middle ear, mastoid antrum, and inner layer of the tympanic membrane.

Second pouch

Contributes to the middle ear, tonsils, supplied by the facial nerve.

Third pouch

The third pouch possesses dorsal and ventral wings. Derivatives of the dorsal wings include the inferior parathyroid glands, while the ventral wings fuse to form the cytoreticular cells of the thymus. The main nerve supply to the derivatives of this pouch is cranial nerve IX, the glossopharyngeal nerve.

Fourth pouch

Derivatives include the superior parathyroid glands and parafollicular C-Cells of the thyroid gland.

Fifth pouch

The rudimentary structure becomes part of the fourth pouch contributing to thyroid C-cells.

Answer 8 – (E) – Branchial cleft 1

The external auditory meatus develops from the first branchial cleft

Answer 9 and Answer 10 – (A) – First branchial arch

The first branchial arch, also called "mandibular arch", develops into...... muscles of mastication, anterior belly of the digastric, mylohyoid, tensor tympani, tensor veli palatini, maxilla, mandible (only as a model for the mandible not the actual formation of mandible), the incus and malleus of the middle ear, also Meckel's cartilage, trigeminal nerve (V2 and V3), and maxillary artery.

Answer 11 and 12 (B) – Second branchial arch

The second branchial arch, also called the "hyoid arch", develops into....... muscles of facial expression, buccinator, platysma, stapedius, stylohyoid, posterior belly of the digastric, stapes, styloid process, hyoid (lesser horn and upper part of body), Reichert's cartilage, facial nerve (VII) and stapedial artery.

Answer 13 – (D) – Genitalia have male/female characteristics

Foetal development in early stages are as follows:

Day 0	Fertilisation
Week 1	Implantation
Week 2	Bilaminar disk
Week 3	Gastrulation, primitive streak, notochord and neural plate begins to form
Week 3–8	Neural tube formed, organogenesis
Week 4	Heart begins to beat. Limb buds begin to form
Week 10	Genitalia have male/female characteristics

Answer 14 (C) – Organogenesis

See above

Answer 15 (A) – Heart begins to beat

See above

Answer 16 – (B) – Captopril

Captopril is an angiotensin converting enzyme which crosses the placental barrier, affects foetal development and inhibits foetal urine production. This foetal anomaly includes renal dysplasia, renal failure, decreases foetal urine production leading to oligohydramnios, hypoplastic calavaria and intrauterine growth retardation.

It is commonly used as an antihypertensive drug.

Answer 17 – (G) – Thalidomide

Thalidomide was sold in a number of countries across the world from 1957 until 1961 when it was withdrawn from the market after being found to be a cause of birth defects in the form of limb defects – "phocomelia".

Thalidomide causes the truncation of limb development by causing loss of newly formed blood vessels as developing limbs are particularly susceptible due to their relatively immature, highly angiogenic vessel network.

It is not known exactly how many worldwide victims of the drug there have been, although estimates range from 10,000 to 20,000.

Thalidomide was found to be a valuable treatment for a number of medical conditions as an effective tranquiliser or painkiller, and was proclaimed as a "wonder drug" for insomnia, coughs, colds and headaches.

It was also found to be an effective antiemetic which had an inhibitory effect on morning sickness. It was a commonly used drug by thousands of pregnant women to relieve their symptoms. At the time of the drug's development it was not thought likely that any drug could pass from the mother across the placental barrier and harm the developing foetus.

Answer 18 – (J) – Diethylstilbestrol

Diethylstilbestrol is a synthetic nonsteroidal estrogen. This was used in prevention of miscarriage a few decades ago. It was found to be associated with clear cell adenocarcinoma of the vagina and cervix.

Answer 19 – (0) – Dark yellow-grey teeth

Tetracycline is a broad spectrum antibiotic which is most commonly used in the treatment of severe acne, chlamydia, syphilis and much other infectious disease. It is a protein synthesis inhibitor. It causes teeth discolouration in the developing foetus as it crosses the placental barrier, therefore it is contraindicated in pregnancy.

Answer 20 – (A) – Surface Ectoderm

The ectoderm is the start of a tissue that covers the body surfaces. It emerges first and forms from the outermost of the germ layers.

The ectoderm differentiates to form the nervous system and the epidermis (the outer part of integument).

In vertebrates, the ectoderm has three parts: external ectoderm (also known as surface ectoderm), the neural crest, and neural tube. The latter two are known as neuroectoderm.

The surface ectoderm (or external ectoderm) forms the following structures:

- Skin (only epidermis as dermis is derived from mesoderm) along with glands, hair and nail

- Epithelium of the mouth and nasal cavity, salivary glands, and glands of mouth and nasal cavity

- Enamel (in teeth) – as a side note dentin and dental pulp are formed from ectomesenchyme which is derived from ectoderm (specifically neural crest cells and with mesenchymal cells)

- Epithelium of pineal and pituitary glands
- Lens and cornea of the eye
- Apical ectodermal ridge inducing development of the limb buds of the embryo
- Sensory receptors in epidermis

Answer 21 – (C) – Neural Crest

The neural crest, a transient component of the ectoderm, located between the neural tube and the epidermis (or the free margins of the neural folds) of an embryo during neural tube formation.

Neural crest cells quickly migrate during or shortly after neurulation, an embryological event marked by neural tube closure.

It has been referred to as the fourth germ layer. The neural crest can give rise to neurons and glia of the autonomic nervous system (ANS); some skeletal elements, tendons and smooth muscle; chondrocytes, osteocytes, melanocytes, chromaffin cells, and supporting cells and hormone producing cells in certain organs.

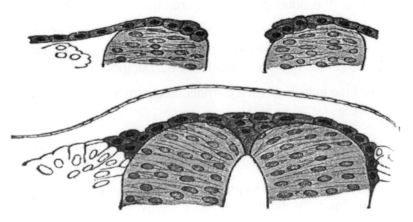

Some derivatives of the neural crest

Derivative	Cell type or structure derived
Peripheral nervous system (PNS)	Neurons, including sensory ganglia, sympathetic and parasympathetic ganglia, and plexuses
	Neuroglial cells
	Schwann cells
Endocrine and paraendocrine derivatives	Adrenal medulla
	Calcitonin-secreting cells
	Carotid body type I cells
Pigment cells	Epidermal pigment cells
Facial cartilage and bone	Facial and anterior ventral skull cartilage and bones
Connective tissue	Corneal endothelium and stroma
	Tooth papillae
	Dermis, smooth muscle, and adipose tissue of skin of head and neck
	Connective tissue of salivary, lacrimal, thymus, thyroid, and pituitary glands
	Connective tissue and smooth muscle in arteries of aortic arch origin

Source: After Jacobson 1991, based on multiple sources.

Answer 22 – (E) – Pseudostratified ciliated columnar

A pseudostratified epithelium is a type of epithelium that, though comprising of only a single layer of cells, has its cell nuclei positioned in a manner suggestive of stratified epithelia.

- Ciliated pseudostratified columnar epithelia are found in the lines of the trachea as well as the upper respiratory tract.

- Non-ciliated pseudostratified columnar epithelia are located in the membranous part of male urethra and vas deferens.

If a specimen looks stratified but has cilia, then it is a pseudostratified ciliated epithelium.

Answer 23 (A) – Non keratinised stratified squamous epithelium

A stratified squamous epithelium consists of squamous (flattened) epithelial cells arranged in layers upon a basement membrane. Only one layer is in contact with the basement membrane; the other layers adhere to one another to maintain structural integrity. Although this epithelium is referred to as squamous, many cells within the layers may not be flattened; this is due to the convention of naming epithelia according to the cell type at the surface.

This type of epithelium is well suited to areas in the body subject to constant abrasion, as the layers can be sequentially sloughed off and replaced before the basement membrane is exposed.

Stratified squamous epithelium is further classified by the presence or absence of keratin at the apical surface. Non-keratinized surfaces must be kept moist by bodily secretions to prevent them drying out and dying, whereas keratinized surfaces are protected from abrasion by keratin and kept hydrated and protected from dehydration by glycolipids produced in the stratum granulosum.

- Non-keratinized stratified squamous epithelium: cornea, oral cavity, oesophagus, rectum, vagina, and the internal portion of the lips.

- Keratinized stratified squamous epithelium: skin, tongue (partially keratinized), and the external portion of the lips

The cervix and vagina are lined by squamous epithelium

Answer 24 – (C) – Non keratinised squamous epithelium

An epithelium is classified as a primary body tissue, connective tissue, muscle tissue and nervous tissue. Primary body epithelial tissue lines the cavities and surfaces of structures throughout the body and also forms many glands. It lies on top of connective tissue, and the two layers are separated by a basement membrane.

Functions of epithelial cells include secretion, selective absorption, protection, transcellular transport and detection of sensation.

Answer 25 – (D) – Ciliated columnar epithelium

The Fallopian tube is the only structure in the female genital tract with a ciliated columnar epithelium; the beating of the cilia helps move the egg into the uterus. This fact is also sometimes clinically helpful since dilated and deformed Fallopian tubes can be microscopically distinguished from cystic ovarian tumours by the presence of the cilia.

Answer 26 – (A) – Autosomal dominant

Osteogenesis imperfecta is an autosomal dominant condition in 80%–90% of cases. It is a recessive condition characterized by bones that break easily, often from little or no apparent cause. Examples of autosomal dominant diseases:

Adult polycystic kidney disease
Achondroplasia
Familial adenomatous polyposis
Familial hypercholesterolemia (Type II A)
Hereditary spherocytosis
Huntington's disease
Marfan's syndrome
Neurofibromatosis
Von Hippel-Lindau disease

Dominant inheritance means an abnormal gene from one parent is capable of causing disease, even though the matching gene from the other parent is normal. The abnormal gene "dominates" the pair of genes. If just one parent has a dominant gene defect, each child has a 50% chance of inheriting the disorder. Dominant inheritance occurs when an abnormal gene from one parent is able to cause disease even though the matching gene from the other parent is normal. The abnormal gene dominates.

For example, if four children are born to a couple and one parent has an abnormal gene for a dominant disease, statistically two children will inherit the abnormal gene and two children will not. Children who do not inherit the abnormal gene will not develop or pass on the disease.

If someone has an abnormal gene that is inherited in an autosomal dominant manner, then the parents should also be tested for the abnormal gene.

Answer 27 – (C) – X-linked recessive

Glucose-6-phosphate dehydrogenase deficiency is X-linked with about 300 variants reported. Most of the variants occur sporadically and are single amino acid defects in a protein of 515 amino acids. G6PD deficiency is an inherited condition in which the body doesn't have enough of the enzyme glucose-6-phosphate dehydrogenase, or G6PD, which helps red blood cells (RBCs) function normally. This deficiency can cause haemolytic anaemia, usually after exposure to certain medications, foods, or even infections.

Any gene located on the X-chromosome is called an X-linked gene. All X-linked genetic conditions, such as G6PD deficiency, are more likely to affect males than females. G6PD deficiency will only manifest itself in females when there are two defective copies of the gene in the genome. As long as there is one good copy of the G6PD gene in a female, a normal enzyme will be produced and this normal enzyme can then take over the function that the defective enzyme lacks. When a certain heritable trait is expressed in such a manner, it is called a recessive trait. In males, however, where there is only one X-chromosome, one defective G6PD gene is sufficient to cause G6PD deficiency

Sex-linked diseases are inherited through one of the "sex chromosomes" – the X or Y chromosomes. X-linked diseases usually occur in males. Males have only one X chromosome. A single recessive gene on that X chromosome will cause the disease.

The Y chromosome is the other half of the XY gene pair in the male. However, the Y chromosome doesn't contain most of the genes of the X chromosome. It therefore doesn't protect the male. This is seen in diseases such as hemophilia and Duchenne muscular dystrophy.

TYPICAL SCENARIOS

For a given birth, if the mother is a carrier (only one abnormal X chromosome) and the father is normal:

- 25% chance of a normal boy
- 25% chance of a boy with disease
- 25% chance of a normal girl
- 25% chance of a carrier girl without disease

If the father has the disease and the mother is normal:

- 100% chance of a normal boy
- 100% chance of a carrier girl without disease

X-Linked recessive disorders in females

Females can get an X-linked recessive disorder, but this is very rare. An abnormal gene on the X chromosome from each parent would be required, since a female has two X chromosomes. This could occur in the two scenarios below.

For a given birth, if the mother is a carrier and the father has the disease:

- 25% chance of a healthy boy

- 25% chance of a boy with the disease
- 25% chance of a carrier girl
- 25% chance of a girl with the disease

If the mother has the disease and the father has the disease:

- 100% chance of the child having the disease, whether boy or girl.

The odds of either of these two scenarios are so low that X-linked recessive diseases are sometimes referred to as "male only" diseases. However, this is not technically correct.

Cystic fibrosis, thalassaemia, Tay-Sachs disease and hereditary haemochromatosis are examples of of autosomal recessive inheritance conditions. Autosomal recessive genetic conditions usually affect men and women equally.

Examples of X-linked recessive diseases :-

Becker's muscular dystrophy, Duchenne muscular dystrophy, Fragile X syndrome; H aemophilia A; Haemophilia B; Red-Green colour blindness; Wiskott-Aldrich syndrome; Lesch-Nyhan syndrome; X-linked agammaglobulinemia

Answer 28 – (B) – Patau syndrome

Patau syndrome is a severe chromosomal abnormality in which the child has an extra chromosome 13. This is usually present in every cell. Unless one of the parents is a carrier of a translocation the chances of a couple having another trisomy 13 affected child is less than 1%. Symptoms of Patau syndrome are:

- mental and motor challenged
- polydactyly (extra digits)
- microcephaly
- low-set ears

- holoprosencephaly (failure of the forebrain to divide properly).

- heart defects

- structural eye defects, including microphthalmia, Peters anomaly, cataract, iris and/or fundus (coloboma), retinal dysplasia or retinal detachment, sensory nystagmus, cortical visual loss, and optic nerve hypoplasia

- cleft palate

- meningomyelocele (a spinal defect)

- omphalocele (abdominal defect)

- abnormal genitalia

- abnormal palm pattern

- overlapping of fingers over thumb

- cutis aplasia (missing portion of the skin/hair)

- prominent heel

- kidney defects

- deformed feet known as "rocker-bottom feet"

Answer 29 – (D) – Turner syndrome

Girls with Turner syndrome are born with only one X chromosome or they are missing part of one X chromosome. The effects of the condition vary widely. It depends on how many of the body's cells are affected by the changes to the X chromosome.

Girls with Turner syndrome are usually short in height. Girls with Turner syndrome who aren't treated for short stature reach an average height of about 4 feet 7 inches (1.4 meters). The good news is that when Turner syndrome is diagnosed while a girl is still growing, she can be treated with growth hormones to help her grow taller.

In addition to growth problems, Turner syndrome prevents the ovaries from developing properly, which affects a girl's sexual development and the ability to have children. Because the ovaries are responsible for making the hormones that control breast growth and menstruation, most girls with Turner syndrome will not go through all of the changes associated with puberty unless they get treatment for the condition. Nearly all girls with Turner syndrome will be infertile, or unable to become pregnant on their own.

In addition to short stature and lack of sexual development, some of the other physical features commonly seen in girls with Turner syndrome are:

- a "webbed" neck (extra folds of skin extending from the tops of the shoulders to the sides of the neck)
- a low hairline at the back of the neck
- drooping of the eyelids
- differently shaped ears that are set lower on the sides of the head than usual
- abnormal bone development (especially the bones of the hands and elbows)
- a larger than usual number of moles on the skin
- oedema

Answer 30 – (A) – Edwards syndrome

Edwards syndrome is trisomy 18, (with an extra chromosome 18 instead of the usual pair).

It is a severe disorder that can affect all organs in the body. It is a very serious abnormality that leads to severe mental and growth retardation, abnormalities in the heart (ventricular septal defect, atrial septal defect, patent ductus arteriosus), and other organs and malformed features that include a small chin, low ears, cleft palate, a webbed neck, and flexed limbs that have deformed hands and feet called arthrogryposis (a muscle disorder that causes multiple joint contractures at birth), kidney malformations, intestines protruding outside the body (omphalocele), oesophageal atresia.

Answer 31 – (D) – Clomophine citrate

Is a selective estrogen receptor modulator (SERM), increasing production of gonadotropins by inhibiting negative feedback on the hypothalamus adverse effect of clomophine include multiple ovulation, hence increasing the chance of twins, ovarian hyperstimulation, wt. gain and ovarain cancer.

Answer 32 – (B) – HRT

Oestrogen causes endometrial proliferation by increasing the number of oestrogen/progesterone receptors, and also increasing the mitotic rate in the glandular cells of the endometrium. Prolonged oestrogenic stimulation is likely to cause progression through increasing degrees of endometrial proliferation to hyperplasia. Endometrial cancer remains a risk for postmenopausal women taking HRT. For over 25 years it has been recognised that unopposed oestrogen is associated with a significant increased risk of endometrial cancer, with relative risks ranging from 1.4 to 12.0, and that this increases with the duration of unopposed therapy up to a relative risk of 15.0

Answer 33 – (C) – Oral contraceptive pills

Oral contraceptives have been shown to increase the risk of cervical cancer; however, human papillomavirus is the major risk factor for this disease.

Oral contraceptive use has been shown in multiple studies to decrease the risk of ovarian and endometrial cancer.

Answer 34 – (A) – Human papillomavirus (HPV) infection

HPV is a necessary factor in the development of nearly all cases of cervical cancer. Types 16 and 18 are generally acknowledged to cause about 70% of cervical cancer cases. Together with type 31, they are the prime risk factors for cervical cancer.

Answer 35 – (D) – EBV

EBV establishes a lifelong dormant infection in some cells of the body's immune system. A late event in a very few carriers of this virus is the emergence of Burkitt's lymphoma and nasopharyngeal carcinoma.

Answer 36 (A) – Primary syphilis

Primary syphilis is typically acquired via direct sexual contact with the infectious lesions of a person with syphilis. Approximately 10–90 days after the initial exposure (average 21 days), a skin lesion appears at the point of contact, which is usually the genitalia, but can be anywhere on the body. This lesion, called a *chancre*, is a firm, painless skin ulceration localized at the point of initial exposure to the spirochete, often on the penis, vagina or rectum. In rare circumstances, there may be multiple lesions present; although it is typical that only one lesion is seen. The lesion may persist for 4 to 6 weeks and usually heals spontaneously. Local lymph node swelling can occur. During the initial incubation period, individuals are otherwise asymptomatic. As a result, many patients do not seek medical care immediately.

Answer 37 – (E) – Genital herpes

It is caused by the herpes simplex virus (HSV). There are two types: HSV-1 and HSV-2. Most genital herpes infections are caused by HSV-2. HSV-1 is the usual cause of what most people call "fever blisters" in and around the mouth and can be transmitted from person to person through kissing. Less often, HSV-1 can cause genital herpes infections through oral sexual contact. The genital sores caused by either virus look the same. Whilst HSV1 is usually associated with cold sores around the mouth and HSV 2 with genital ulcers, in practice each virus can cause both types of symptom.

Answer 38 – (H) – Anti-dsDNA

Systemic lupus erythematosus (SLE) is a multiorgan system autoimmune disease with numerous immunological and clinical manifestations. It is characterized by an autoantibody response to nuclear and cytoplasmic antigens

(A) Anti-DNA: Antibody to native DNA in abnormal titer *or*

(B) Anti-Sm: Presence of antibody to Sm nuclear antigen

(C) Positive finding of antiphospholipid antibodies based on (1) an abnormal serum level of IgG or IgM anticardiolipin antibodies, (2) a positive test result for lupus anticoagulant using a standard method, or (3) a false-positive serologic test for syphilis known to be positive for at least 6 months and confirmed by *Treponema pallidum* immobilization or fluorescent treponemal antibody absorption tests *or* Antinuclear antibody: An abnormal titer of antinuclear antibody by immunofluorescence or an equivalent assay at any point in time and in the absence of drugs known to be associated with drug-induced lupus syndrome

Answer 39 – (G) – Anti-epithelial cell antibodies

Pemphigus vulgaris is associated with anti-epithelial cell antibodies. This condition is characterised by painful intra-epidermal bullae and superficial vesicles that present on the skin and mucosa. The diagnosis is confirmed by a skin biopsy. The autoimmune response against the intercellular antigen results in suprabasilar acantholysis. A sensitive but nonspecific clinical sign seen in PV is Nikolsky's sign, referring to the separation of the superficial epidermal layers from the basal layer on exertion of tangential pressure over perilesional skin Asboe-Hansen sign, where compressing an intact bulla forces fluid to spread under the skin away from the site of pressure.

Answer 40 – (A) – Genomic imprinting

The distinction of chromosome by paternal origin is due to imprinting and PWS has the sister syndrome Angelman syndrome that affects maternally imprinted genes in the region It is characterized by hypotonia, short stature, polyphagia, obesity, small hands and feet, hypogonadism, and mild mental retardation.

Answer 41 – (E) – Multifactorial inheritance

Type 1 diabetes appears to be triggered by some (mainly viral) infections, with some evidence pointing at Coxsackie B4 virus. There is a genetic element in individual susceptibility to some of these triggers which has been traced to particular HLA genotypes (i.e., the genetic "self" identifiers relied upon by the immune system). However, even in those who have inherited the susceptibility, type 1 diabetes mellitus seems to require an environmental trigger. First-degree relatives with type 2 have a much higher risk of developing type 2, (increasing with the number of those relatives). Concordance among monozygotic twins is close to 100%, and about 25% of those with the disease have a family history of diabetes. Moreover, obesity (which is an independent risk factor for type 2 diabetes) is strongly inherited. Monogenic forms, e.g., MODY, constitute 1–5 % of all cases.

Answer 42 – (H) – Mitochondrial inheritance

Leber hereditary optic neuropathy is caused by mutations in mt DNA and is transmitted by maternal inheritance. It is characterized by bilateral, painless, subacute visual failure that develops during young adult life. Affected individuals are usually entirely asymptomatic until they develop visual blurring affecting the central visual field in one eye; similar symptoms appear in the other eye an average of eight weeks later. In an estimated 25% of cases, visual loss is bilateral at onset. Visual acuity is severely reduced to counting fingers or worse in most cases, and visual field testing shows an enlarging central or centrocecal scotoma.

Answer 43 – (E) – PCR

PCR allows isolation of DNA fragments from genomic DNA by selective amplification of a specific region of DNA. This use of PCR augments many methods, such as generating hybridization probes for southern or northern hybridization and DNA cloning, which require larger amounts of DNA, representing a specific DNA region. PCR supplies these techniques with high amounts of pure DNA, enabling analysis of DNA samples even from very small amounts of starting material.

Answer 44 – (A) – Southern blot

Southern blot is a method routinely used in molecular biology for detection of a specific DNA sequence in DNA samples. Southern blotting combines transfer of electrophoresis-separated DNA fragments to a filter membrane and subsequent fragment detection by probe hybridization.

Answer 45 – (B) – Internal iliac lymph nodes

They surround the internal iliac artery and its branches, and receive the lymphatics corresponding to the distribution of the branches of it, i. e., they receive lymphatics from all the pelvic viscera, from the deeper parts of the perineum, including the membranous and cavernous portions of the urethra, and from the buttock and back of the thigh.

Answer 46 – (C) – External iliac lymph nodes

They lie along the external iliac vessels. Their principal afferents are derived from the inguinal lymph nodes, the deep lymphatics of the abdominal wall below the umbilicus and of the adductor region of the thigh, and the lymphatics from the glans penis vel clitoridis, the membranous urethra, the prostate, the fundus of the urinary bladder, the cervix uteri, and upper part of the vagina.

Answer 47(C) – The caval opening is at T8

The IVC is formed by the joining of the left and right common iliac veins and brings blood into the right atrium of the heart. It also anastomoses with the azygos vein system and the venous plexuses next to the spinal cord.

The specific levels of the tributaries are as follows:

Vein	Level
inferior phrenic vein	T8
hepatic vein	T8
suprarenal veins	L1
renal veis	L1
gonadal vein	L2
lumbar veins	L1–L5
common iliac vein	L5

Answer 48 (E) – T10

The oesophagus is a muscular tube of 25 cm length (connecting pharynx & stomach). It is flattened anteroposteriorly. It begins in the neck at the lower border of cricoid cartilage, level of C6 vertebra, piercing the diaphragm at the level of vertebra T10 and ends by opening in to the stomach at the level of vertebra T11.

Answer 49 (G) – T12

The aorta begins at the level of the diaphragm, crossing it via the aortic hiatus, technically behind the diaphragm, at the vertebral level of T12.

It travels down the posterior wall of the abdomen in front of the vertebral column. It thus follows the curvature of the lumbar vertebrae, that is, convex anteriorly. The peak of this convexity is at the level of the third lumbar vertebra (L3)

Answer 50 – (K) – Tracheal bifurcation occurs at T4.

The trachea has an inner diameter of about 20 to 25 millimetres (0.79 to 0.98 in) and a length of about 10 to 16 centimetres (3.9 to 6.3 in). It commences at the larynx, level with the fifth cervical vertebra, and bifurcates into the primary bronchi at the vertebral level of T4/T5.

Answer 51 (E) – Neisseria

They are Gram-negative bacteria included among the proteobacteria, a large group of Gram-negative forms. *Neisseria* are diplococci that resemble coffee beans when viewed microscopically. Different *Neisseria* species can be identified by the sets of sugars from which they will produce acid. For example, *N. gonorrheae* makes acid from only glucose, however *N. meningitidis* produces acid from both glucose and maltose.

Answer 52 (D) – Clostridium spp.

They are obligate anaerobes capable of producing endospores. Individual cells are rod-shaped. *C. botulinum*, an organism producing a toxin in food/wounds that causes botulism. *C. difficile*, which can overgrow other bacteria in the gut during antibiotic therapy, can cause pseudomembranous colitis. *C. perfringens* – gas gangrene. *C. tetani*, the causative organism of tetanus.

Answer 53 (T) – Non-gonococcal urethritis

It is an inflammation of the urethra which is not caused by gonorrheal infection. *C. trachomatis* is an obligate intracellular pathogen (i.e. the bacterium lives within human cells) and can cause numerous disease states in both men and women. Both sexes can display urethritis, proctitis (rectal disease and bleeding), trachoma, and infertility. The bacterium can cause prostatitis and epididymitis in men. In women, cervicitis, pelvic inflammatory disease (PID), ectopic pregnancy, and acute or chronic pelvic pain are frequent complications. *C. trachomatis* is also an important neonatal pathogen, where it can lead to infections of the eye (trachoma) and pulmonary complications.

Answer 54 (G) – Mesenteric Adenitis

Gram-negative bacillus that belongs to the family Enterobacteriaceae. is most frequently associated with acute diarrhea, terminal ileitis, mesenteric lymphadenitis, and pseudoappendicitis.

Answer 55 (N) – Q fever

The causative organism for Q fever is C burnetii. This is a strict, intracellular, pleomorphic, gram-negative coccobacillus classified as a Legionellales species. The primary means of infection in Q fever are inhalation of aerosolized organisms during occupational exposure, exposure to parturient animals, and from tick bites.

Answer 56 (I) – Plague

The classic mode of transmission to humans is a flea bite. The incubation period of plague is 3–4 days. *Y pestis* is a nonmotile, pleomorphic, gram-negative coccobacillus that belongs to the family Enterobacteriaceae. Bipolar staining (giving the appearance of a closed safety pin) can be observed with Giemsa, Wayson, or Wright stains.

Answer 57 (K) – Influenza

Vaccines containing killed microorganisms - these are previously virulent micro-organisms which have been killed with chemicals or heat. Examples are vaccines against flu, cholera, bubonic plague, polio and hepatitis A

Answer 58 (G) – Hepatitis B

Recombinant vaccines are those in which genes for desired antigens are inserted into a vector, usually a virus,that has a very low virulence. The vector expressing the antigen may be used as the vaccine, or the antigen may be purified and injected as a subunit vaccine.

The only recombinant vaccine currently in use in humans is the Hepatitis B Virus (HBV) vaccine, which is a recombinant subunit vaccine.

Hepatitis B surface antigen is produced from a gene transfected into yeast cells and purified for injection as a subunit vaccine. This is much safer than using attenuated HBV, which could cause lethal hepatitis or liver cancer if it reverted to its virulent phenotype

Answer 59 (B) – Immunoglobulin A (IgA)

It is an antibody which plays a critical role in mucosal immunity. IgA is the main immunoglobulin found in mucous secretions, including tears, saliva, colostrum and secretions from the genitourinary tract, gastrointestinal tract, prostate and respiratory epithelium.

Answer 60 (A) – IgG

IgG molecules are synthesised and secreted by plasma B cells. Constituting 75% of serum immunoglobulins, this is the only isotype that can pass through the human placenta, thereby providing protection to the foetus in utero. Along with IgA secreted in the breast milk, residual IgG absorbed through the placenta provides the neonate with humoural immunity before its own immune system develops.

Answer 61 (C) – Asbestos

Mesothelioma is almost always caused by exposure to asbestos. Its most common site is the pleura. It may also occur in the peritoneum, the heart, the pericardium or tunica vaginalis.

Answer 62 (F) – Aniline dyes

Smoking is the most commonly associated risk factor and accounts for approximately 50% of all bladder cancers. Nitrosamine, 2-naphthylamine, and 4-aminobiphenyl are possible carcinogenic agents found in cigarette smoke. Bladder cancer is also associated with industrial exposure to aromatic amines in dyes, paints, solvents, leather dust, inks, combustion products, rubber, and textiles.

Answer 63 (C) – Addison's disease

Addison's disease is adrenocortical insufficiency due to the destruction or dysfunction of the entire adrenal cortex. It affects glucocorticoid and mineralocorticoid function. Effects – hyperpigmentation of the skin and mucous membranes, progressive weakness, fatigue, poor appetite, and weight loss, dizziness with orthostasis due to hypotension. Myalgias and flaccid muscle paralysis may occur due to hyperkalemia.

Answer 64 (R) – Carcinoid syndrome

Carcinoid tumours are of neuroendocrine origin and derived from primitive stem cells, which can give rise to multiple cell lineages. Appendicular carcinoid tumours are most common, producing the vasoactive substance, serotonin. The most important clinical finding is flushing of the skin, usually of the head and the upper part of thorax. Secretory diarrhoea and abdominal cramps are also characteristic features of the syndrome. Other associated symptoms are nausea, and vomiting. Bronchoconstriction affects a smaller number of patients and often accompanies flushing.

Answer 65 (J) – Scleroderma

It is classically defined as symmetrical skin thickening, with about 90% of cases also presenting with Raynaud's phenomenon, nail-fold capillary changes, anti-nuclear antibodies and occasionally by biopsy. Of the antibodies, 90% have a detectable anti-nuclear antibody.

Answer 66 (B) Ribosomes

They are the workhorses of protein biosynthesis, the process of translating mRNA into protein. The mRNA comprises a series of codons that dictate to the ribosome the sequence of the amino acids needed to make the protein.

Answer 67 (A) Mitochondria

The most prominent roles of mitochondria are to produce ATP (i.e., phosphorylation of ADP) through respiration, and to regulate cellular metabolism.

Answer 68 (I) Microtubules

They are one of the components of the cytoskeleton. Microtubules serve as structural components within cells and are involved in many cellular processes including mitosis, cytokinesis, and vesicular transport.

Answer 69 (F) Porphyrin

The key precursor to porphyrins is biosynthesized from glycine, which provides the central subunit of all purines. Glycine is an inhibitory neurotransmitter in the central nervous system, especially in the spinal cord, brainstem, and retina.

Answer 70 (A) Epinephrine

Phenylalanine can also be converted into L-tyrosine, another one of the DNA-encoded amino acids. L-tyrosine in turn is converted into L-DOPA, which is further converted into dopamine, norepinephrine and epinephrine.

Answer 71 (A) Vitamin B1

Thiamine is a water-soluble vitamin of the B complex (vitamin B_1). Nerve cells and other supporting cells (such as glial cells) of the nervous system require thiamine. Examples of neurologic disorders that are linked to alcohol abuse include Wernicke's encephalopathy (WE, Wernicke-Korsakoff syndrome) and Korsakoff's psychosis (alcohol amnestic disorder) as well as varying degrees of cognitive impairment. It also causes wet and dry beriberi.

Answer 72 (A) Same as above

Answer 73 (C) Vitamin B3

Niacinamide is one of the water-soluble B-complex vitamins. Niacin, or nicotinic acid, is also known as Vitamin B-3. Symptoms include muscular weakness, general fatigue, irritability, dizziness, loss of appetite, headaches, swollen red tongue, skin lesions including rashes, dry scaly skin in areas exposed to sunlight, wrinkles, coarse skin texture, nausea and vomiting and its late symptoms include dementia and death.

Answer 74 (F) Vitamin B12

Deficiency causes megaloblastic anaemia, and sub acute combined degeneration of the spinal cord.

Answer 75 (A) Frequency used in diagnostic ultrasound is 1–10 MHz.

Diagnostic sonography (ultrasonography) is an ultrasound-based diagnostic imaging technique used to visualize subcutaneous body structures including tendons, muscles, joints, vessels and internal organs for possible pathology or lesions. Obstetric sonography is commonly used during pregnancy and is widely recognized. Typical diagnostic sonographic scanners operate in the frequency range of 2 to 18 megahertz, hundreds of times greater than the limit of human hearing. The choice of frequency is a trade-off between spatial resolution of the image and imaging depth: lower frequencies produce less resolution but image deeper into the body.

Answer 76 (J) – Cobalt-60

It is a radioactive metal that is used in radiotherapy. It produces two gamma rays. Cobalt-60 has a radioactive half-life of 5.27 years. This decrease in activity requires periodic replacement of the sources used in radiotherapy and is one reason why cobalt machines have been largely replaced by linear accelerators in modern radiation therapy. Cobalt from radiotherapy machines has been a serious hazard when not disposed of properly.

Answer 77 (F) Alpha particles

Named after and denoted by the first letter in the Greek alphabet, they consist of two protons and two neutrons bound together into a particle identical to a helium nucleus. They are a highly ionizing form of particle radiation, and have low penetration depth. Alpha particles are commonly emitted by all of the larger radioactive nuclei such as uranium, thorium, actinium, and radium, as well as the transuranic elements.

Answer 78 (Q) 1J/kg

The gray (symbol: Gy) is the SI unit of absorbed radiation dose due to ionizing radiation (for example, X-rays). One *gray* is the absorption of one joule of energy, in the form of ionizing radiation, by one kilogram of matter.

The gray measures the deposited energy of radiation. The biological effects vary by the type and energy of the radiation and the organism and tissues involved. This SI unit is named after Louis Harold Gray.

Answer 79 (A) Vasopressin

Arginine vasopressin (AVP), also known as vasopressin, argipressin or antidiuretic hormone (ADH), is synthesized in the hypothalamus and stored in vesicles at the posterior pituitary. Most of it is stored in the posterior pituitary to be released into the blood stream. Water excretion by the kidney is regulated by the peptide hormone vasopressin. Vasopressin increases the water permeability of the renal collecting duct cells, allowing more water to be reabsorbed from collecting duct urine to blood.

Answer 80 (B) – Aldosterone

It is a steroid hormone (mineralocorticoid family) produced by the outer-section (zona glomerulosa) of the adrenal cortex in the adrenal gland, and acts on the distal tubules and collecting ducts of the kidney to cause the conservation of sodium, secretion of potassium, increased water retention, and increased blood pressure. The overall effect of aldosterone is to increase reabsorption of ions and water in the kidney.

Answer 81 (E) – Calcitonin

It is produced by the parafollicular cells (also known as C-cells) of the thyroid. It acts to reduce blood calcium (Ca^{2+}), opposing the effects of parathyroid hormone (PTH). It inhibits Ca^{2+} absorption by the intestines, osteoclast activity in bones, phosphate reabsorption by the kidney tubules and increases absolute Ca^{2+} and Mg^+ reabsorption by the kidney tubules. Calcitonin is a renal Ca-conserving hormone.

Answer 82 (O) Pulmonary fibrosis

The drug is used in the treatment of Hodgkin lymphoma (as a component of the ABVD regimen), squamous cell carcinomas, and testicular cancer, as well as in the treatment of pleurodesis. The most serious complication of bleomycin is pulmonary fibrosis and impaired lung function. Other side effects include fever, rash, dermatographism, hyperpigmentation, alopecia and Raynaud's phenomenon

Answer 83 (G) Gynaecomastia

Spironolactone is a potassium sparing diuretic. It inhibits the effect of aldosterone by competing for intracellular aldosterone receptors in the distal convoluted tubule cells. This decreases the reabsorption of sodium and water, while decreasing the secretion of potassium. The adverse effects include hyperkalemia, gynaecomastia, menstrual irregularities and testicular atrophy.

Answer 84 (F) Agranulocytosis

Clozapine is an atypical antipsychotic drug adverse effects include agranulocytosis, cardiac toxicity, gastrointestinal hypo motility, weight gain and diabetes.

Answer 85 (I) Nephrotoxicity and ototoxicity

Amino glycosides are protein synthesis inhibitors which act on the 30S ribosomal unit used in severe gram negative infections. Its adverse effects include nephrotoxicity and ototoxicity.

Answer 86 (A) Osteoporosis

Long-term corticosteroids use has several severe side effects as for example: hyperglycemia, insulin resistance, diabetes mellitus, osteoporosis, anxiety, depression, gastritis, colitis, hypertension, ictus, erectile dysfunction, hypogonadism, hypothyroidism, amenorrhoea and retinopathy.

Answer 87 (C) Diabetes insipidus

Lithium carbonate is used as a mood stabiliser for bipolar disorder; it blocks relapse and acute manic events. Its mechanism is possibly related to phosphoinositol cascade. Its adverse effects include tremors, hypothyroidism, and nephrogenic diabetes insipidus.

Answer 88 (F) Dopamine

It is produced in several areas of the brain, including the substantia nigra and the ventral tegmental area. Dopamine is also a neurohormone released by the hypothalamus. Its main function as a hormone is to inhibit the release of prolactin from the anterior lobe of the pituitary.

Answer 89 (K) GH

GH also stimulates production of insulin-like growth factor 1 (IGF-1, formerly known as somatomedin C), a hormone homologous to proinsulin. The liver is a major target organ of GH for this process and is the principal site of IGF-1 production. IGF-1 has growth-stimulating effects on a wide variety of tissues. Additional IGF-1 is generated within target tissues, making it appear to be both an endocrine and an autocrine/paracrine hormone. IGF-1 also has stimulatory effects on osteoblast and chondrocyte activity to promote bone growth.

Answer 90 (M) Oxytocin

Oxytocin is made in magnocellular neurosecretory cells of the supraoptic and paraventricular nuclei of the hypothalamus and is stored in Herring bodies at the axon terminals in the posterior pituitary. It is then released into the blood from the posterior lobe (neurohypophysis) of the pituitary gland. Oxytocin acts at the mammary glands, causing milk to be 'let down' into a collecting chamber, from where it can be extracted by compressing the areola and sucking at the nipple. It causes uterine contractions during the second and third stages of labour.

Answer 91 (G) – LH

LH is a hormone produced by the anterior pituitary gland. In the *female*, an acute rise of LH – the *LH surge* – triggers ovulation and corpus luteum development and in the male it stimulates Leydig cell production of testosterone.

Answer 92 (J) Clomophine citrate

Clomophine is a selective estrogen receptor modulator (SERM), increasing production of gonadotropins by inhibiting negative feedback on the hypothalamus. It is used mainly for ovarian stimulation in female infertility due to anovulation. Adverse effects of clomophine include multiple ovulation, hence increasing the chance of twins, ovarian hyperstimulation, weight gain and ovarian cancer.

Answer 93 (D) Goserelin

Goserelin acetate (Zoladex,) is an injectable gonadotropin releasing hormone super-agonist (GnRH agonist), also known as a lutenizing hormone releasing hormone (LHRH) agonist. Goserelin acetate is used to treat hormone-sensitive cancers of the prostate and breast (in pre-/perimenopausal women) and some benign gynaecological disorders (endometriosis, uterine fibroids and endometrial thinning).

Answer 94 (A) Rosiglitazone

It is an anti-diabetic drug in the thiazolidinedione class of drugs used as a mono or in combination with other diabetic drugs. It acts by increasing target cell response to insulin.

Answer 95 (E) Finasteride

Finasteride is a 5-alpha reductase inhibitor which decreases the conversion of testosterone to dihydrotestosterone. Used for the treatment of benign prostatic hypertrophy and also used to treat male pattern baldness.

Answer 96 (H) Ascorbic acid

The L-enantiomer of ascorbic acid is also known as vitamin C. The name "ascorbic" comes from its property of preventing and curing scurvy. Ascorbate acts as an antioxidant by being available for energetically favourable oxidation and plays a primary role in collagen formation which is essential for the growth and repair of tissue cells, gums, blood vessels, bones. Ascorbic acid has been found to be specifically required for the decarboxylation of alpha-ketoglutarate in the prolyl-4-hydroxylase reaction, where it may act as a compound necessary for the reduction of enzyme-bound ferric iron formed during proline hydroxylation.

Answer 97 (K) Tocopherol

Tocopherol (Vitamin E) is the most important lipid-soluble antioxidant, in that it protects cell membranes from oxidation by reacting with lipid radicals produced in the lipid peroxidation process.

Answer 98 (F) Cobalamin

In patients biochemically deficient for cobalamin, methylmalonic acid (MMA) is increased in the serum and urine, but normalizes after treatment with vitamin B12. With vitamin B12 deficiency, the conversion of L-methylmalonyl-Co-A to succinyl-Co-A is reduced, and is instead metabolized to methylmalonic acid. A more sensitive method of screening for vitamin B_{12} deficiency is measurement of serum methylmalonic acid and homocysteine levels

Answer 99 (I) Retinol

Vitamin A is also called retinol. Vitamin A is required in the production of rhodopsin, the visual pigment used in night vision.

Answer 100 (J) Pseudomonas aeruginosa

It is a Gram-negative, aerobic rod belonging to the bacterial family Pseudomonadaceae. The bacterium almost never infects uncompromised tissues, yet there is hardly any tissue that it cannot infect if the tissue defences are compromised in some manner. It causes urinary tract infections, respiratory system infections, dermatitis, soft tissue infections, bacteraemia, bone and joint infections, gastrointestinal infections and a variety of systemic infections (particularly in patients with severe burns and in cancer and AIDS patients who are immunosuppressed). Produces pyocyanin (blue green pigment), endotoxin and exotoxin A.

Answer 101 (D) HIV

HIV is a retrovirus. It is a single stranded linear RNA virus whose capsule symmetry is icosahedral.

Answer 102 (I) Trichomonas vaginalis

Is an anaerobic, parasitic flagellated protozoan, is the causative agent of trichomoniasis. *T. vaginalis* trophozoite is oval as well as flagellated. *T. vaginalis* was traditionally diagnosed via a wet mount, in which "corkscrew" motility was observed. Infection is treated and cured with metronidazole or tinidazole, and should be prescribed to any sexual partner(s) as well because they may potentially be asymptomatic carriers.

Answer 103 (H) Treponema pallidum

Syphilis is a venereal disease caused by infection with the spirochete *Treponema pallidum.*

T pallidum is able to cross the placenta in pregnant women and result in foetal infection. Untreated syphilis progresses through 4 stages: primary, secondary, latent, and tertiary.

Answer 104 (A) RSV

RSV is a single-stranded RNA virus of the family *Paramyxoviridae*, which includes common respiratory viruses such as those causing measles and mumps. Nearly all children will have been infected with the virus by 2–3 years of age. Treatment is supportive care only with fluids and oxygen until the illness runs its course.

Answer 105 (E) E. coli

E. coli is a Gram-negative, facultative non-sporulating anaerobic and it is the most common cause of UTI.

Harmless strains of *E. coli* can be found widely in nature, including the intestinal tracts of humans and warm-blooded animals. Disease-causing strains, however, are a frequent cause of both intestinal and urinary-genital tract infections.

The urinary tract is the most common site of *E coli* infection, and more than 90% of all uncomplicated UTIs are caused by *E coli* infection. The recurrence rate after a first *E coli* infection is 44% over 12 months. *E coli* UTIs are caused by uropathogenic strains of *E coli* which cause a wide range of UTIs, including uncomplicated urethritis/cystitis, symptomatic cystitis, pyelonephritis, and urosepsis. Uncomplicated cystitis occurs primarily in females who are sexually active and are colonized by an uropathogenic strain of *E coli*. Subsequently, the periurethral region is colonized from contamination of the colon, and the organism reaches the bladder during sexual intercourse.

Answer 106 (I) Legionella

It is a Gram negative bacterium, and includes species that cause legionellosis or Legionnaires' disease. Common sources include cooling towers, domestic hot-water systems, fountains, and similar disseminators that tap into a public water supply. It can survive in temperatures up to 55 °C.

Answer 107 (H) HBV

Transmission of hepatitis B virus results from exposure to infectious blood or body fluids containing blood. Possible forms of transmission include (but are not limited to) unprotected sexual contact, blood transfusions, re-use of contaminated needles and syringes, and vertical transmission from mother to child during childbirth.

Answer 108 (D) HCG

The subunit of human chorionic gonadotropin is also secreted by some cancers including choriocarcinoma, germ cell tumours, hydatidiform mole formation, teratoma with elements of choriocarcinoma (this is rare), and islet cell tumour.

Answer 109 (I) TRAP

It is highly expressed by osteoclast, activated macrophages, neurons, and the porcine endometrium during pregnancy. There are also certain pathological conditions in which expression of TRAP is increased. These include patients with leukaemic reticuloendotheliosis (hairy cell leukaemia), Gaucher's disease, HIV-induced encephalopathy, osteoclastoma and osteoporosis, and metabolic bone diseases.

Answer 110 (C) Alpha-fetoprotein

It is a normal foetal serum protein synthesized by the liver, yolk sac, and gastrointestinal tract that shares sequence homology with albumin. It is a major component of foetal plasma, reaching a peak concentration of 3 mg/ml at 12 weeks of gestation. AFP is a marker for hepatocellular and germ cell (nonseminoma) carcinoma.

Answer 111 (M) Acute lymphoblastic leukaemia

Children with Down's syndrome (DS) are at increased risk of both acute lymphoblastic leukaemia (ALL) and acute myeloid leukaemia (AML).

Answer 112 (H) Adenocarcinoma of the oesophagus

Barrett's oesophagus is marked by the presence of columnar epithelia in the lower oesophagus, replacing the normal squamous cell epithelium—an example of metaplasia. The secretory columnar epithelium may be more able to withstand the erosive action of the gastric secretions; however, this metaplasia confers an increased risk of adenocarcinoma

Answer 113 (D) Osteosarcoma

Paget's disease is associated with the development of osteogenic sarcoma. When there is a sudden onset or worsening of pain, sarcoma should be considered. Osteogenic sarcoma is an extremely rare complication that occurs in less than one percent of all patients.

Answer 114 (J) Cardiac rhabdomyoma

Tuberous sclerosis affects tissues from different germ layers. Cutaneous and visceral lesions may occur, including adenoma sebaceum, cardiac rhabdomyomas, and renal angiomyolipomas.

Answer 115 (C) Kaposi's sarcoma

It is a tumour caused by human herpes virus 8 (HHV8), it is one of the AIDS defining illnesses.

KS lesions are nodules or blotches that may be red, purple, brown, or black, and are usually papular (i.e. palpable or raised).

They are typically found on the skin, but internal location elsewhere is common, especially the mouth, gastrointestinal tract and respiratory tract. Growth can range from very slow to explosively fast, and is associated with significant mortality and morbidity.

Answer 116 (B) Thymoma

Up to 75% of patients have an abnormality of the thymus; 25% have a thymoma, a tumour (either benign or malignant) of the thymus, and other abnormalities are frequently found. The disease process generally remains stationary after thymectomy (removal of the thymus).

Answer 117 (B) Phenothiazine

The phenothiazine structure occurs in various neuroleptic drugs, e.g. chlorpromazine, and antihistaminic drugs, e.g. promethazine.

The term "phenothiazines" describes the largest of the five main classes of neuroleptic antipsychotic drugs. These drugs have antipsychotic and, often, antiemetic properties, although they may also cause severe side effects such as akathisia, tardive dyskinesia, extrapyramidal symptoms, and the rare but potentially fatal neuroleptic malignant syndrome as well as substantial weight gain.

Answer 118 (H) Protease inhibitors

They are a class of medications used to treat or prevent infection by viruses, including HIV and Hepatitis C. They prevent viral replication by inhibiting the activity of HIV-1 protease.

Answer 119 (G) Tricyclic antidepressants (TCAs)

TCAs inhibit the reabsorption (reuptake) of serotonin and norepinephrine by brain cells. To a lesser extent, TCAs also inhibit reabsorption of dopamine. Examples include Amitriptyline, Amoxapine, Desipramine, Doxepin Imipramine, Nortriptyline, Protriptyline, Trimipramine.

Answer 120 (M) Methylxanthines

They are a group of alkaloids commonly used for their effects as mild stimulants and as bronchodilators, notably in treating the symptoms of asthma. Methylated xanthine derivatives include caffeine, paraxanthine, theophylline, and theobromine. These drugs act as both non-selective phosphodiesterase inhibitors and adenosine receptor antagonists.

Answer 121 (G) Same as 119

Answer 122 (D)

Metabolic acidosis results from either an excess of acid or reduced buffering capacity due to a low concentration of bicarbonate. Excess acid may occur due to increased production of organic acids or, more rarely, ingestion of acidic compounds.

Answer 123 (E)

Metabolic alkalosis results from the excessive loss of hydrogen ions, the excessive reabsorption of bicarbonate or the ingestion of alkalis. It is a condition in which the pH of the blood is elevated beyond the normal range (7.35–7.45). This is usually the result of decreased hydrogen ion concentration, leading to increased bicarbonate, or alternatively a direct result of increased bicarbonate concentrations.

Answer 124 (B)

Respiratory acidosis results when the $PaCO_2$ is above the upper limit of normal, >6kPa (45mmHg). It is most commonly due to decreased alveolar ventilation causing decreased excretion of CO_2. Less commonly it is due to excessive production of CO_2 by aerobic metabolism.

Answer 125 (C)

Respiratory alkalosis results from the excessive excretion of CO_2, and occurs when the $PaCO_2$ is less than 4.5kPa. This is commonly seen in hyperventilation due to anxiety states.

Answer 126 (C) Type III hypersensitivity

Type III hypersensitivity is also known as immune complex hypersensitivity. The reaction may be general (e.g., serum sickness) or may involve individual organs including skin (e.g., systemic lupus erythematosus, Arthus reaction), kidneys (e.g., lupus nephritis), lungs (e.g., aspergillosis), blood vessels (e.g., polyarteritis), joints (e.g., rheumatoid arthritis) or other organs. This reaction may be the pathogenic mechanism of diseases caused by many microorganisms.

Answer 127 (C) same as above

Answer 128 (D) Type IV hypersensitivity

Also known as cell mediated or delayed type hypersensitivity. The classical example of this hypersensitivity is tuberculin (Montoux) reaction which peaks 48 hours after the injection of antigen (PPD or old tuberculin). The lesion is characterized by induration and erythema. Mechanisms of damage in delayed hypersensitivity include T lymphocytes and monocytes and/or macrophages. Cytotoxic T cells (Tc) cause direct damage whereas helper T (TH1) cells secrete cytokines which activate cytotoxic T cells and recruit and activate monocytes and macrophages, which cause the bulk of the damage.

Answer 129 (A) Sensitivity = true positive/all people with disease. High sensitivity is desirable for a screening test.

Answer 130 (B) Specificity = true negative/all people without disease. High specificity is desirable for a confirmatory test.

Answer 131 (A) The volume of urine present in the bladder after normal voiding is 0–10 ml.

Answer 132 (B) Normal urine flow in an adult female is with a peak flow rate of 25 ml/sec. Flow rates are highest and more predictable with 200–400 ml urine volume.

Answer 133 (K) Normal bladder capacity is approximately 550–600 ml.

Answer 134 (M) Normal voiding pressure is 45–70 cm of water.

Answer 135 (G) 1 gram of carbohydrate = **4 Cal**.

Carbohydrate is a short-term energy store consisting of simple sugars which are absorbed in 5 to 10 minutes (eg table sugar), and long-chain complex molecules which can take up to an hour to digest (eg starch in plants, maltodextrin in energy drinks). Carbohydrate is stored in muscles as glycogen.

Answer 136 (F) The energy value per gram of fat – **37kJ (9 Cal)**

Animal studies show that polyunsaturated, mono-unsaturated and saturated fatty acids are broken down differently in the body and may not be used in the same way. Some fats, like polyunsaturated fats (especially omega-3 fatty acids from fish oils), may be more easily used up from fat stores during exercise than fats from other animal sources. This suggests that saturated fat may be more likely to go into and stay in fat cells than some forms of polyunsaturated fat and possibly mono-unsaturated fat.

Answer 137 (G) 1 gram of protein = 4 Cal.

Protein should account for 10% to 20% of the calories consumed each day. Protein is essential to the structure of red blood cells, for the proper functioning of antibodies resisting infection, for the regulation of enzymes and hormones, for growth, and for the repair of body tissue.

Answer 138 (G) Mitochondria

They are cellular power plants, and are also involved in a range of other processes, such as signalling, cellular differentiation, cell death, as well as the control of the cell cycle and cell growth.

Answer 139 (D) Golgi apparatus

The primary function of the Golgi apparatus is to process and package macromolecules, such as proteins and lipids, after their synthesis and before they make their way to their destination; it is particularly important in the processing of proteins for secretion.

Answer 140 (C) Lysosomes

They are the cells' garbage disposal system. They are used for the digestion of macromolecules from phagocytosis, endocytosis, and autophagy. Other functions include digesting foreign bacteria that invade a cell and helping repair damage to the plasma membrane.

Answer 141 (F) Ribosomes

They are the workhorses of protein biosynthesis, carrying out the process of translating mRNA into protein.

Answer 142 (F) HBeAg

Hepatitis B e-antigen (HBeAg): A positive (or reactive) result indicates the presence of virus that can be passed to others. A negative result usually means the virus cannot be spread to others.

A strong correlation was found between HBeAg positivity of the serum of hepatitis B surface antigen (HBsAg) carrier women and the subsequent development of surface antigenaemia in their babies. All babies who became chronic HBsAg carriers were born to HbeAg positive women. Maternal HBeAg positivity being a better prior indication of chronic antigenaemia developing in the baby than the HBsAg titer in the mother's serum.

HBeAg is a viral protein associated with HBV infections. Unlike the surface antigen, the e-antigen is found in the blood only when there are viruses also present. HBeAg is often used as a marker of ability to spread the virus to other people (infectivity). Measurement of e-antigen may also be used to monitor the effectiveness of HBV treatment; successful treatment will usually eliminate HBeAg from the blood and lead to development of antibodies against e-antigen (anti-HBe).

Answer 143 (C) HBsAb

The *hepatitis B surface antibody (anti-HBs) is* the most common test. Its presence indicates previous exposure to HBV, but the virus is no longer present and the person cannot pass on the virus to others. The antibody also protects the body from future HBV infection. In addition to exposure to HBV, the antibodies can also be acquired from successful vaccination. This test is done following the completion of vaccination against the disease or following an active infection.

Answer 144 (B) HBsAg

HBsAg antibody confers life-long immunity and the presence of HBeAg indicates low transmissibility.

Answer 145 (E) HBCaB

Anti-hepatitis B core antigen (anti-HBc) is an antibody to the hepatitis B core antigen. The core antigen is found on virus particles but disappears early in the course of infection. This antibody is produced during and after an acute HBV infection and is usually found in chronic HBV carriers as well as those who have cleared the virus, and usually persists for life.

Answer 146 (A) Haemophilia A

Is the most common type of haemophilia. It is also known as factor VIII deficiency or classic haemophilia. It is largely an inherited disorder in which one of the proteins needed to form blood clots is missing or reduced. In about 30% of cases, there is no family history of the disorder and the condition is the result of a spontaneous gene mutation.

Answer 147 (B) Haemophilia B

is the second most common type of haemophilia. It can also be known as factor IX deficiency, or Christmas disease. By and large, haemophilia B tends to be similar to haemophilia A but less severe.

Answer 148 (E) Bernard-Soulier disease

An inherited human platelet disorder, is characterized by decreased adhesion of platelets to the subendothelium. It is a rare inherited bleeding disorder caused by abnormal platelets and subsequent abnormal clotting. It is one of the giant platelet syndromes. This is referred to as an adhesion complex and forms a receptor that enables platelets to stick together to form a clot. It is also called haemorrhagiparous thrombocytic dystrophy, a rare autosomal recessive coagulopathy (bleeding disorder), and is characterised by prolonged bleeding time, thrombocytopenia, giant platelets, and decreased platelet survival.

Answer 149 (B) Immunoglobulin A (IgA)

is an antibody which plays a critical role in mucosal immunity. More IgA is produced in mucosal linings than all other types of antibody. IgA is the main immunoglobulin found in mucous secretions, including tears, saliva, colostrum and secretions from the genito-urinary tract, gastrointestinal tract, prostate and respiratory epithelium.

Answer 150 (A) IgG

IgG is the only isotype that can pass through the human placenta, thereby providing protection to the foetus in utero. Along with IgA secreted in the breast milk, residual IgG absorbed through the placenta provides the neonate with humoural immunity before its own immune system develops. Colostrum contains a high percentage of IgG.

Immunoglobulin G (IgG) is a monomeric immunoglobulin, built of two heavy chains and two light chains. Each IgG has two antigen binding sites. It is the most abundant immunoglobulin and is approximately equally distributed in blood and in tissue liquids, constituting 75% of serum immunoglobulins in humans.

Answer 151 (B) Osteosarcoma

It is known that patients affected by hereditary Rb have 1000 times the incidence of osteosarcoma compared with the general population. Sporadic osteosarcomas show alteration of the Rb gene in 70% of cases. Abnormalities of the Rb gene are commonly seen in osteosarcoma but other components of the RB-pathway gene can be subject to genetic alterations.

Osteosarcoma is a malignant neoplasm of bone. It is among the most common non haematologic primary malignant tumours of bone in both children and adults. The conventional type arises in the intramedullary cavity of the bone and represents 75% of all osteosarcomas. These tumours penetrate and destroy the cortex of the bone and extend into surrounding soft tissues. In conventional intramedullary osteosarcoma, the predominant histologic pattern may be osteoblastic, fibroblastic, chondroblastic, giant cell rich, malignant fibrous histiocytoma-like or partially telangiectatic.

Answer 152 (G) Breast cancer

BRCA1 is a breast cancer susceptibility gene that was first identified in 1994. People carrying a mutation (abnormality) in this gene are at an increased risk of breast or ovarian cancer. The normal gene plays a role in repairing breaks in DNA. However, when the gene is mutated it is thought that this repair function may become disabled thus leading to more DNA replication errors and cancerous growth.

Answer 153 (F) Li-Fraumeni syndrome

LFS is a rare autosomal dominant hereditary disorder. The syndrome increases greatly the susceptibility to cancer. The syndrome is linked to germline mutations of the p53 tumour suppressor gene, which normally helps control cell growth. Mutations can be inherited or can arise de novo early in embryogenesis or in one of the parent's germ cells. Persons with LFS are at risk for a wide range of malignancies, with particularly high occurrences of breast cancer, brain tumours, acute leukemia, soft tissue sarcomas, bone sarcomas, and adrenal cortical carcinoma.

Answer 154 (G) ErbB2

The ErbB2/Neu/HER2 oncogene is amplified and overexpressed in 20%–30% of human breast cancer cases, and expression of ErbB2 is associated with aggressive metastatic tumour behaviour, decreased time to clinical relapse and poor prognosis. ErbB2 is overexpressed in 25%–30% of breast and ovarian cancers, correlates with poor prognosis and lower survival and has also been associated with chemoresistance. Transfection of erbB2 resulted in cells stably overexpressing the protein and showing increased motility compared to the empty vector control cells.

Answer 155 (F) RET

Multiple endocrine neoplasia type 2 (MEN2) is an inherited, autosomal-dominant disorder caused by deleterious mutations within the *RET* protooncogene. MEN2 *RET* mutations are mainly heterozygous, missense sequence changes found in *RET* exons 10, 11, and 13–16.

Multiple endocrine neoplasia type 2 (also known as Sipple's Syndrome) is a group of medical disorders associated with tumours of the endocrine system. The tumours may be benign or malignant (cancer). They generally occur in endocrine organs (e.g. thyroid, parathyroid, and adrenals), but may also occur in endocrine tissues of organs not classically thought of as endocrine.

Answer 156 (C) c-myc

Over expression of c-myc is one of the most common alterations in human cancers, yet it is not clear how this transcription factor acts to promote malignant transformation. The consistent appearance of specific chromosomal translocations in human Burkitt lymphomas and murine plasmacytomas has suggested that these translocations might play a role in malignant transformation. Transformation of these cells is frequently accompanied by the somatic rearrangement of a cellular analogue of an avian retrovirus transforming gene, c-myc. The oncogene *c-myc* is frequently associated with human malignancies and plays a critical role in regulating cell proliferation, growth, apoptosis, and differentiation.

Answer 157(G) Thayer-Martin agar

(or **Thayer-Martin medium**) is a Mueller-Hinton agar with 5% chocolate agar, sheep blood and antibiotics. It is used for culturing and primarily isolating pathogenic *Neisseria* bacteria, including *Neisseria gonorrhoeae* and *Neisseria meningitidis*, as the medium inhibits the growth of most other microorganisms.

Answer 158 (H) Chocolate agar with factor V and X

Bacterial culture of *H. influenzae* is performed on nutrient agar, preferably Chocolate agar, plate with added X(Hemin) & V(NAD) factors at 37°C in an enriched CO_2 incubator.

Answer 159 (D) Lowenstein-Jensen medium

LJ medium, is a growth medium specially used for culture of Mycobacterium, notably *Mycobacterium tuberculosis*.

Answer 160 (F) Ziehl-Neelsen stain

Also known as the acid-fast stain. It is a special bacteriological stain used to identify acid-fast organisms, mainly mycobacteria.

Answer 161 (B) Congo red

It is used to stain microscopic preparates, especially as a cytoplasm and erythrocyte stain. Apple-green birefringence of Congo red stained preparates under polarized light is indicative for the presence of amyloid fibrils. Congo red is used as a sensitive diagnosis tool for amyloidosis, instead of the traditional histological birefringence test.

Answer 162 (E) India ink

It facilitates the visualization of cryptococcal polysaccharide capsules. The capsular material of cryptococci displaces the colloidal carbon particles of the ink so that the capsule appears as a clear halo around the microorganisms against a black background.

Answer 163 (B) Cholecystokinin

It is synthesised by I-cells in the mucosal epithelium of the small intestine and secreted in the duodenum, the first segment of the small intestine, and causes the release of digestive enzymes and bile from the pancreas and gallbladder, respectively.

Answer 164 (F) Pepsin

Pepsin is an enzyme that is released by the chief cells in the stomach and that degrades food proteins into peptides.

Answer 165 (A) Proximal convoluted tubule

The proximal tubule as a part of the nephron can be divided into an initial convoluted portion and a following straight (descending) portion. Fluid in the filtrate entering the proximal convoluted tubule is reabsorbed into the peritubular capillaries, including approximately two-thirds of the filtered salt and water and all filtered organic solutes (primarily glucose and amino acids).

Answer 166 (E) Collecting tubule

It can reabsorb or secrete sodium, potassium, hydrogen, and ammonium ions depending on the body's requirements; it also reabsorbs some water in the filtrate and secretes urea.

Answer 167 (A) HDL

HDL plays a major role in reverse cholesterol transport, mobilizing cholesterol from the periphery to promote return to the liver. In the general population, lower-than-normal HDL cholesterol levels are closely correlated with coronary heart disease (CHD); the risk of a coronary event is thought to increase 2% for every 1% decrease in HDL cholesterol.

Answer 168 (D) Chylomicrons

They are formed in the intestine and transport dietary triglyceride to peripheral tissues and cholesterol to the liver. The enzyme lipoprotein lipase, with apolipoprotein (apo)C-II as a co- factor, hydrolyzes chylomicron triglyceride, allowing the delivery of free fatty acids to muscle and adipose tissue.

Answer 169 (G) Internal iliac artery

The uterine artery usually arises from the anterior division of the internal iliac artery (formerly known as the **hypogastric artery**). It is the main artery of the pelvis.

Answer 170 (D) Abdominal aorta

The ovarian artery arises from the abdominal aorta below the renal artery, and does not pass out of the abdominal cavity.

Answer 171 (G) Internal iliac artery

The internal pudendal artery is an artery that branches off the internal iliac artery, providing blood to the external genitalia. It is the terminal branch of the anterior trunk of the internal iliac artery. It is smaller in the female than in the male.

Answer 172 (I) Anterior lobe of pituitary

The anterior pituitary, also called the adenohypophysis, is the glandular, anterior lobe of the pituitary gland. The anterior pituitary regulates several physiological processes including stress, growth, and reproduction. Gonadotrophs, which amount to about 7 percent of all pituitary cells, secrete two hormones, luteinizing hormone (LH) and follicle-stimulating hormone (FSH), but not in equal amount. The rate of secretion varies widely at different ages and at different times in the menstrual cycle of the female.

Answer 173 (J) Posterior lobe of pituitary

The posterior lobe stores and releases two hormones, oxytocin and vasopressin, from nerve cells in specialized regions of the hypothalamus that control pituitary function. These hormones stimulate uterine contraction and milk secretion (oxytocin), and blood pressure and fluid balance (vasopressin).

Answer 174 (C) Beta cells of pancreas

They are a type of cell in the pancreas in areas called the islets of Langerhans. They make up 65–80% of the cells in the islets.

Answer 175 (F) Liver

Cholecalciferal is hydroxylated to 25-hydroxycholecalciferol by the enzyme 25-hydroxylase within the liver. Vitamin D, as either

D_3 or D_2, does not have significant biological activity. It must be metabolized within the body to the hormonally-active form known as 1,25-dihydroxycholecalciferol.

Answer 176 (H) Lung

Angiotensin-converting enzyme (ACE) plays a central role in generating angiotensin II from angiotensin I, and capillary blood vessels in the lung are one of the major sites of ACE expression and angiotensin II production in the human body.

Answer 177 (B) Zona glomerulosa

It constitutes 15% of the adrenal cortex (lying just underneath the capsule), secretes aldosterone (which is the principal mineral corticoid), and contains the enzyme aldosterone synthesis which is necessary for the synthesis of aldosterone.

The secretion of these cells is controlled mainly by the extra cellular fluid concentration of angiotensin II and potassium, both of which stimulate aldosterone secretion.

Answer 178 (D) Fragile X syndrome

It is a genetic condition involving changes in part of the X chromosome. It is the most common form of inherited mental retardation in males and a significant cause of mental retardation in females. Symptoms are the following

- Hyperactive behaviour
- Large body size
- Large forehead or ears with a prominent jaw
- Large testicles (macro-orchidism) after the beginning of puberty
- Mental retardation
- Tendency to avoid eye contact

Answer 179 (F) Osteogenesis imperfecta

OI is a genetically determined disorder of connective tissue characterized by bone fragility. The disease state encompasses a phenotypically and genotypically heterogeneous group of inherited disorders that result from mutations in the genes that code for type I collagen. The disorder is manifest in tissues in which the principal matrix protein is type I collagen (mainly bone, dentin, sclerae, and ligaments).

Answer 180 (H) Sickle cell disease

SCD is a heterogeneous disorder, with clinical manifestations including chronic haemolysis, an increased susceptibility to infections and vaso-occlusive complications often requiring medical care. Patients with SCD can develop specific and sometimes life-threatening complications, as well as extensive organ damage reducing both their quality of life and their life expectancy.

Answer 181 (E) Thymoma

In adults myesthenia gravis is 10 times more frequent than Lambert-Eaton syndrome but it is sometimes difficult to distinguish the 2 disorders, clinically and electromyographically. In adults with MG there is at least a 20% occurrence of thymoma or other neoplasm.

Answer 182 (H) Renal cell carcinoma

One to five percent of human renal cell carcinomas are associated with polycythemia. It is generally assumed that polycythemia results from the secretion of erythropoietin (Epo) by the malignant cells. However, there is no direct proof supporting this hypothesis.

Answer 183 (A) Small cell carcinoma of lung

Excess production of certain hormones by the adrenal gland can lead to symptoms such as weight gain, weakness, and high blood pressure. This is caused by cancer cells (small cell lung carcinoma) making ACTH, a hormone that causes the adrenal glands to secrete cortisol. Secretion of ectopic adrenocorticotropic hormone (ACTH) with consequently Cushing's syndrome is a rare paraneoplastic phenomenon.

Answer 184 (J) Pernicious anaemia

It is a condition where vitamin B12 cannot be absorbed. It is the most common cause of vitamin B12 deficiency in the UK. It is due to an 'autoimmune disease'. Antibodies are formed against intrinsic factor, or against the cells in the stomach which make intrinsic factor. It is thought that something triggers the immune system to make antibodies against intrinsic factor.

Answer 185 (B) – Hereditary spherocytosis

It is a genetically-transmitted disease characterized by the production of red blood cells that are sphere-shaped rather than doughnut-shaped, and therefore more prone to haemolysis. Spectrin deficiency is the most common deficiency found. It is heterogeneous in terms of clinical expression, inheritance (dominant or recessive) and underlying genetic defects.

Answer 186 (C) – Sickle-cell disease

Sickle cell disease or sickle-cell anaemia is a life-long blood disorder characterized by red blood cells that assume an abnormal, rigid, sickle shape. Sickle-cell anaemia is caused by a point mutation in the ß-globin chain of haemoglobin, replacing the amino acid glutamic acid with the less polar amino acid valine at the sixth position of the ß chain. Sickling occurs because of a mutation in the haemoglobin gene. Life expectancy is shortened, with studies reporting an average life expectancy of 42 and 48 years for males and females, respectively.

Answer 187 (D) Mitochondrial inheritance

The inheritance of a trait encoded in the mitochondrial genome. Persons with a mitochondrial disease may be male or female but they are always related in the maternal line and no male with the disease can transmit it to his children.

Answer 188 (G) Anticipation

In genetics, anticipation is a phenomenon whereby the symptoms of a genetic disorder become apparent at an earlier age as it is passed on to the next generation. In most cases, an increase of severity of symptoms is also noted. Anticipation is common in trinucleotide repeat disorders such as Huntington's disease and myotonic dystrophy where a dynamic mutation in DNA occurs. All of these diseases have neurological symptoms.

Answer 189 (C) X-linked recessive

X linked diseases are single gene disorders that reflect the presence of defective genes on the X chromosome. This chromosome is present as two copies in females but only as one copy in males.

The inheritance patterns of X-linked diseases in family pedigrees are complicated by the fact that males always pass their X chromosome to their daughters but never to their sons, whereas females pass their X chromosomes to daughters and sons equally.

Answer 190 (D) Occipital lobe

The occipital lobe is the visual processing centre of the mammalian brain containing most of the anatomical region of the visual cortex.

Answer 191 (C) Parietal lobe

It is a lobe in the brain positioned above the occipital lobe and behind the frontal lobe. Its role is to integrate sensory information from different modalities, particularly determining spatial sense and navigation.

Answer 192 (F) Thalamus

The thalamus is a midline paired symmetrical structure within the brain. It is situated between the cerebral cortex and midbrain, both in terms of location and neurological connections. Its function includes relaying sensation, special sense and motor signals to the cerebral cortex, along with the regulation of consciousness, sleep and alertness.

Answer 193 (C) Thymine

Thymine is one of the four nucleobases in the nucleic acid of DNA that are represented by the letters G–C–A–T. The others are adenine, guanine, and cytosine.

DNA double helix is stabilized by hydrogen bonds between the bases attached to the two strands. Thymine combined with deoxyribose creates the nucleoside deoxythymidine, which is synonymous with the term thymidine. These four bases are attached to the sugar/phosphate to form the complete nucleotide, as shown for adenosine monophosphate.

Answer 194 (E) Uracil

It is a common and naturally occurring pyrimidine derivative. RNA is very similar to DNA, but differs in a few important structural details: in the cell, RNA is usually single-stranded, while DNA is usually double-stranded; RNA nucleotides contain ribose while DNA contains deoxyribose; and RNA has the base uracil rather than thymine that is present in DNA.

Answer 195 (C) S

In the S phase, the chromosomes containing the genetic code (DNA) are copied so that both of the new cells formed will have matching strands of DNA. S phase lasts about 18 to 20 hours.

Answer 196 (E) G0

Resting phase is a period in the cell cycle where the cell has not yet started to divide, a quiescent state. Cells spend much of their lives in this phase. Depending on the type of cell, G0 can last for a few hours to a few years. When the cell gets a signal to reproduce, it moves into the G1 phase.

Answer 197 (D) β_2

Activation of β_2-adrenoceptors in the lungs causes bronchodilation. β_2-adrenoceptor activation leads to hepatic glycogenolysis and pancreatic release of glucagon, which increases plasma glucose concentrations. β_1-adrenoceptor stimulation in the kidneys causes the release of renin, which stimulates the production of angiotensin II and the subsequent release of aldosterone by the adrenal cortex.

Answer 198 (C) β_1

Actions of the β_1 receptor include increased cardiac output, heart rate, atrial cardiac muscle contractility, renin release from juxtaglomerular cells, and lipolysis in adipose tissue.

Answer 199 (L) H2

Gastric acid secretion happens in several steps. Chloride and hydrogen ions are secreted separately from the cytoplasm of parietal cells and mixed in the canaliculi. Gastric acid is then secreted into the lumen of the oxyntic (parietal) gland and gradually reaches the main stomach lumen.

Answer 200 (D)

Osteoporosis is a systemic skeletal disease characterized by low bone mass and micro-architectural deterioration of bone tissue, with a consequent increase in bone fragility and susceptibility to bone fracture. Alkaline phosphatase, calcium, and phosphate levels are normal.

Answer 201 (C)

Vitamin D intoxication can result in hypercalcaemia, raised phosphate and alkaline phosphatase in blood.

Answer 202 (A)

In cases of primary hyperparathyroidism or tertiary hyperparathyroidism serum calcium is increased due to:

1. increased bone resorption, allowing flow of calcium from bone to blood

2. reduced renal clearance of calcium

3. increased intestinal calcium absorption

Serum phosphate: In primary hyperparathyroidism, serum phosphate levels are abnormally low as a result of decreased renal tubular phosphate reabsorption.

Alkaline phosphatase levels do not increase in primary hyperparathyroidism but may increase in secondary hyperparathyroidism.

Answer 203 (L) Tricyclic antidepressant

Amitriptyline is a tricyclic antidepressant. They are a class of psychoactive drugs which is approved for the treatment of major depression. They are named after their chemical structure, which contains three rings of atoms. The "tetracyclic antidepressants" (TeCAs), which contain four rings of atoms, are a closely related group that is often grouped together with the tricyclics, because clinically these drugs are primarily classified by their effect upon receptors.

Answer 204 (L) Tricyclic antidepressant

Imipramine was the first tricyclic antidepressant developed. It was first tried against psychotic disorders, such as schizophrenia, but proved insufficient. During the clinical studies, its antidepressant qualities were unsurpassed by other antidepressants. It is often considered the "gold standard" antidepressant, because its ability to lift the most severe depressive episodes is good.

Answer 205 (E) Benzodiazepine

Diazepam is a benzodiazepine with CNS depressant properties and a somewhat flatter dose-response slope than the sedative-hypnotic drugs. It is relatively devoid of autonomic effects and does not significantly reduce locomotor activity at low doses, or depress amphetamine-induced excitation. In high doses, it activates the drug metabolizing enzymes in the liver. Diazepam also possesses dependence liability and may produce withdrawal symptoms, but has a wide margin of safety against poisoning.

Answer 206 (C) Barbiturate

Phenobarbitone is a barbiturate. It is the most widely used anticonvulsant worldwide and the oldest still commonly used. It also has sedative and hypnotic properties but, as with other barbiturates, has been superseded by the benzodiazepines for these indications. It is recommended as first-line use for partial and generalized tonic-clonic seizures (those formerly known as Grand Mal) in developing countries.

Answer 207 (K) Phenothiazine

Chlorpromazine is an aliphatic phenothiazine. Phenothiazines are thought to elicit their antipsychotic and antiemetic effects via interference with central dopaminergic pathways. Extrapyramidal side effects are a result of interaction with dopaminergic pathways in the basal ganglia.

Chlorpromazine increases prolactin secretion due to its dopamine receptor blocking action in the pituitary and hypothalamus causing galactorrhea and gynaecomastia.

Answer 208 (A) Hypokalaemia

It is a metabolic disorder brought on by potassium deficiency, in which the potassium level in blood is low.

ECG patterns seen in patients with hypokalaemia range from slight T-wave flattening alone to the appearance of prominent U waves. The U wave becomes taller in hypokalaemia which may signify decreased potassium levels in the blood. When the U wave is greater than the T wave, the potassium level is usually less than 2.7 mEq per L (2.7 mmol per L).

The most common causes of hypokalaemia are medications

(especially diuretics) or renal loss related to metabolic alkalosis or potassium loss in the stool secondary to diarrhoea.

Answer 209 (C) Ventricular repolarisation

VR duration, increased transmural dispersion of repolarization (TDR) and early after depolarizations (EAs) are the three electrophysiological components generating the high risk of ventricular arrhythmias and sudden death in the inherited long-QT syndrome (LQT). In the most prevalent LQT1 form of LQT, treatment with beta-blockers reduces serious arrhythmia events dramatically without a known influence on QT interval duration.

Answer 210 (F) Atrial depolarisation

The P wave represents the wave of depolarisation that spreads from the SA node throughout the atria. The brief isoelectric (zero voltage) period after the P wave represents the time in which the impulse is traveling within the AV node (where the conduction velocity is greatly retarded) and the bundle of His. The atrial rate can be calculated by determining the time interval between P waves. P R interval represents the time between the onset of atrial depolarisation and the onset of ventricular depolarisation.

Answer 211 (C) Functional Reserve Capacity

FRC is the volume of air present in the lungs at the end of passive expiration. At FRC, the elastic recoil forces of the lungs and chest wall are equal but opposite and there is no exertion by the diaphragm or other respiratory muscles. FRC is the sum of Expiratory Reserve Volume (ERV) and Residual Volume (RV)

Answer 212 (H) Residual volume

RV is the volume of air remaining in the lungs at the end of a maximal expiration. Air remaining in the lungs after the most complete expiration possible; it is elevated in diffuse obstructive emphysema and during an attack of asthma. Also known as residual air.

Answer 213 (F) Tidal volume

Tidal volume is the volume of air inspired or expired with each normal breath, normally about 500 ml. The amount of air breathed in or out during normal respiration.

Answer 214 (G) Expiratory reserve volume

Expiratory reserve volume (ERV) refers to the extra volume of air that can be exhaled with maximum effort beyond the level reached at the end of a normal, passive exhalation.

Answer 215 (K) L4

The deep tendon reflexes provide information on the integrity of the central and peripheral nervous system. Generally, decreased reflexes indicate a peripheral problem, and lively or exaggerated reflexes a central one.

- Biceps reflex (C5, C6)
- Brachioradialis reflex (C5, C6, C7)
- Extensor digitorum reflex (C6, C7)
- Triceps reflex (C6, C7, C8)
- Patellar reflex or knee-jerk reflex (L2, L3, L4)
- Ankle jerk reflex (Achilles reflex) (S1, S2)
- Plantar reflex or Babinski reflex (L5, S1, S2)

Answer 216 (C) C5 see above

Answer 217 (M) S1 see above

Answer 218 (E) C7 see above

Answer 219 (F) C8 and T1 nerve injury

Klumpke's paralysis is a form of paralysis involving the muscles of the forearm and hand, resulting from a brachial plexus injury in which the eighth cervical (C8) and first thoracic (T1) nerves are injured either before or after they have joined to form the lower trunk. The subsequent paralysis affects, principally, the intrinsic muscles of the hand and the flexors of the wrist and fingers. The injury can result from difficulties in childbirth. The most common aetiological mechanism is caused by a traumatic vaginal delivery, necessitated by shoulder dystocia.

Answer 220 (D) C5 and C6 nerve injury

Erb-Duchenne Palsy is a paralysis of the arm caused by injury to the upper group of the arm's main nerves, specifically, spinal roots C5–C7. These form part of the brachial plexus, comprising the ventral rami of spinal nerves C5–C8, and T1. These injuries arise most commonly from shoulder dystocia during a difficult birth.

Answer 221 (F) Patent ductus arteriosus

A continuous machine-like murmur in the upper left sternal border is common with patent ductus arteriosus (PDA). This is a persistence of the foetal connection (ductus arteriosus) between the aorta and pulmonary artery after birth, resulting in a left-to-right shunt. Symptoms may include failure to thrive, poor feeding, tachycardia, and tachypnoea.

Answer 222 (A) Aortic stenosis

The murmur of aortic stenosis is typically a mid-systolic ejection murmur, heard best over the "aortic area" or right second intercostal space, with radiation into the right neck. This radiation is such a sensitive finding that its absence should cause the physician to question the diagnosis of aortic stenosis. It has a harsh quality and may be associated with a palpably slow rise of the carotid upstroke.

Answer 223 (B) Aortic regurgitation

The hallmark of aortic regurgitation/insufficiency is a high-pitched decrescendo diastolic murmur at the left sternal border after the second heart sound. An Austin-Flint murmur, which is caused by the regurgitant flow causing vibration of the mitral apparatus, is lower pitched and short in duration. The decrescendo diastolic murmur is heard best with the patient leaning forward in full expiration in a quiet room. It is the cardiac murmur most commonly missed.

Answer 224 – (H) X-linked recessive

Haemophilia is an X linked recessive disorder with the following characteristics

- only males are affected
- heterozygous females are clinically unaffected but carry the mutant gene
- rarely will a female manifest the signs of an X-linked disease; this is usually due to atypical lyonization (X-inactivation), a new mutation in the other X chromosome, a carrier with Turner's syndrome, or X-autosome translocation. Female carriers may inherit the defective gene from either their mother, father, or it may be a new mutation
- milder signs of X-linked disorders may evolve in the female due to normal lyonization.

The following are the most frequently encountered X-linked recessive conditions:

- red-green colour blindness
- fragile X-linked mental retardation
- non-specific X-linked mental retardation
- Duchenne muscular dystrophy
- Becker muscular dystrophy
- Haemophilia A (factor VIII)

- Haemophilia B (factor IX)
- X-linked ichthyosis
- X-linked agammaglobulinaemia

Answer 225 (I) Mitochondrial inheritance

Leber's hereditary optic neuropathy (LHON) or Leber optic atrophy is a mitochondrially inherited (mother to all offspring) degeneration of retinal ganglion cells (RGCs) and their axons that leads to an acute or subacute loss of central vision; this affects predominantly young adult males. However, LHON is only transmitted through the mother as it is primarily due to mutations in the mitochondrial (not nuclear) genome and only the egg contributes mitochondria to the embryo.

Answer 226 (A) Autosomal dominant

Huntington's chorea is inherited in an autosomal dominant pattern located on chromosome 4, which means one copy of the altered gene in each cell is sufficient to cause the disorder. Child of an affected parent has a 50% risk of inheriting the disease. In rare situations where both parents have an affected gene, and either parent has two affected copies, this risk is greatly increased. Physical symptoms of Huntington's disease begin at any age from infancy to old age, but usually begin between 35 and 44 years of age. On rare occasions, when symptoms begin before about 20 years of age, they progress faster and vary slightly. Huntington's disease is a progressive brain disorder that causes uncontrolled movements, emotional problems, and loss of thinking ability (cognition).

Answer 227 (L) Rubella

This is a classic presentation of Rubella (measles), specially the pathognomonic (Koplic spots). It seldom has an effect on the unborn baby in mid trimester. Vaccination is not indicated during pregnancy and of no value if already infected.

Answer 228 (B) Chlamydia trachomatis

The infant is likely to have caught *C. Trachomatis* conjunctivitis from his/her mother. Diagnosis can be confirmed by immunologic enzyme assay.

Answer 229 (O) Calymmatobacterium granulomatis

This is a typical presentation of donovanosis (granuloma inguinale), caused by calymmato-bacterium granulomatis. It is a sexually transmitted disease with 1–12 weeks incubation period. It presents as coalescing, ulcerating, nodules that may not be painful unless secondary infection has occurred. The pathognomonic Donovan bodies are dark staining. It is treated with tetracyclines.

Answer 230 (C) – Treponema pallidum

Primary syphilis is associated with painless genital ulcers (chancre) on the labia, vulva, vagina, cervix, anus, lips or nipples. The lesion appears 10 to 90 days after the initial infection. The chancre lasts 1 to 5 weeks and will resolve without treatment but the infective organism remains. The disease is treated with penicillin, erythromycin or tetracycline.

Answer 231 (P) Cytomegalovirus

Cytomegalovirus is an asymptomatic maternal infection, which can be passed to the foetus. Nearly all infected babies are asymptomatic at birth. The virus can be isolated from any body fluid.

Answer 232 (J) Mycobacterium tuberculosis

Tuberculosis can cause PID and infertility. Diagnosis with endometrial biopsy is consistent with late disease stage and surgery is often required because of failed antibiotic treatment.

Answer 233 (C) Medroxy progesterone injectable contraception

LARC "Long acting reversible contraception" includes the following alternatives:- Intrauterine device (IUD), Mirena Intrauterine system (IUS), contraceptive implant (Implanon), Depo-Provera injection. Note – oestrogen containing contraceptives cannot be used in patients with migraine.

Answer 234 (G) LNG – Intra Uterine System (Mirena)

The progesterone component is helpful in the treatment of menorrhagia by causing atrophy of the endometrium and has the added contraception benefit.

Answer 235 (D) Condoms (male and female)

A condom is one of the main contraceptive methods that give protection against STIs, however it has a high failure rate.

Answer 236 (N) Levonorgestrel 1.5 mg

High dose progesterone is effective up to 72 hours after unprotected intercourse with Levnorgestrel given in 0.75 mg in two divided doses 12 hours apart or 1.5 mg given as one dose.

Answer 237 (H) Female Sterilisation

It is important to inform patients about the failure rate of each contraception method in sterilisation. it is necessary to mention 1:200 life time risk not HWY (Hundred Woman Years).

Answer 238 (E) Secondary postpartum haemorrhage

Secondary PPH is defined as any bleeding from the genital tract after 24 hours of delivery (retained products or clots as major cause). Secondary infection or sepsis may be present in the PPH.

Answer 239 (J) Placenta praevia

Typical presentation is p/v bleeding associated without any abdominal pain which could be provoked by intercourse. Placenta praevia exists when the placenta is inserted wholly or in part into the lower segment of the uterus. Symptomatic placenta praevia is associated with the sudden onset of painless bleeding in the second or third trimester. Women with placenta praevia are reported to be 14 times more likely to bleed in the antenatal period compared with women without placenta praevia.

Answer 240 (C) Placenta abruption (Abruptio placenta)

Wooden hard abdomen with haemodynamic as well as p/v bleeding is typical presentation of placental abruption, which is a recognised complication of severe pre-eclampsia.

Answer 241 (G) In labour

This patient is presenting with normal labour, it is common to have blood stained show with cervical dilatation.

Answer 242 (G) Transvaginal USS of the pelvis, Pipelle biopsy

Postmenopausal bleeding warrants prompt investigations to exclude endometrial cancer. The role of the transvaginal scan is to measure the endometrial thickness and check any mass or lesion. The role of pipelle biopsy is to detect any abnormality with endometrial histopathology.

Answer 243 (D) Laparotomy

Patient is haemodynamically unstable therefore there is no time practically to do laparoscopy. It is better to do laparotomy in these situations to avoid unnecessary delay.

Answer 244 (J) Diagnostic laparoscopy and dye injection

Initial assessment of tubal function is important to assess the reason for her primary subfertility. Diagnostic laparoscopy may help in the diagnosis of her endometriosis as shown by her symptoms.

Answer 245 (C) Colposcopy and directed biopsy

Colposcopy aids magnifications and directed biopsy of the lesion, which is suggestive of cervical cancer.

Answer 246 (G) 25% of children will be affected and 75% will be normal

Autosomal dominant so there is a 50% chance the woman has inherited the achondroplasia gene. If she has, then there is a 50% chance of passing the gene on to any one of her children. So the probability of any child being affected is 50% × 50% = 25%, leaving 75% normal.

Answer 247 (J) 50% of children will be carriers and 50% will be affected

Autosomal recessive. The woman is the carrier, the partner has got the disease.

Answer 248 (C) 50% of boys will be affected and 50% of girls will be carriers.

In X-linked inheritance, male offspring are always affected, females are carriers.

Answer 249 (A) All children will be affected

As of the balanced translocation, this woman's gametes will be either forming zygotes with monosomy 21 which is not compatible with life or with trisomy 21 so all children will have Down's syndrome.

Answer 250 (B) Gestational diabetes mellitus

The two main risks GDM imposes on the baby are growth abnormalities and chemical imbalances after birth, which may require admission to a neonatal intensive care unit. Infants born to mothers with GDM are at risk of being large for gestational age (macrosomic). Macrosomia in turn increases the risk of instrumental delivery (e.g. forceps, ventouse and caesarean section).

Answer 251 (K) Cholestasis of pregnancy

Obstetric cholestasis is a condition of the liver which occurs in some pregnant women. Cholestasis means there is a reduced flow of bile down the bile ducts in the liver. Some bile then 'leaks' out into the bloodstream, in particular the bile salts. These circulate in the bloodstream and can cause symptoms. The main symptom is persistent itch in the later third of pregnancy.

Answer 252 (H) Pulmonary embolism

Venous thromboembolism (VTE) refers to the formation of a thrombus within veins. This can occur anywhere in the venous system but the clinically predominant sites are in the vessels of the leg (giving rise to deep vein thrombosis, DVT) and in the lungs (resulting in a pulmonary embolus, PE). The pathophysiology of VTE in pregnancy appears to relate to the increased venous stasis noted during this period but other factors such as alterations in the balance of proteins of the coagulation and fibrinolytic systems have also been implicated. Its importance in obstetrics is highlighted by the statistic that PE is the most common cause of maternal death in the UK.

Answer 253 (M) HELLP Syndrome

HELLP syndrome is a life-threatening obstetric complication usually considered to be a variant of pre-eclampsia. Both conditions occur during the later stages of pregnancy. HELLP is an abbreviation of the main findings: Haemolytic anaemia, Elevated Liver enzymes and Low Platelet count.

Answer 254 (B) Gestational diabetes mellitus

GDM is a condition in which women without previously diagnosed diabetes exhibit high blood glucose levels during pregnancy.

Gestational diabetes generally has few symptoms and it is most commonly diagnosed by screening during pregnancy. Diagnostic tests detect inappropriately high levels of glucose in blood samples. Gestational diabetes affects 3–10% of pregnancies, depending on the population studied. No specific cause has been identified, but it is believed that the hormones produced during pregnancy increase a woman's resistance to insulin, resulting in impaired glucose tolerance.

Babies born to mothers with gestational diabetes are at increased risk of problems, such as being large for gestational age (which may lead to delivery complications), low blood sugar, and jaundice. It is a treatable condition and women who have adequate control of glucose levels can effectively decrease these risks.

Answer 255 (F) Meigs' syndrome

The three cardinal features of Meigs' syndrome are: benign ovarian tumour, ascites and pleural effusion. If the tumour is resected, the fluid resolves. The ovarian tumour is usually a fibroma but may be a thecoma, cystadenoma, or granulosa cell tumour. When the histology is other than fibroma, it is sometimes referred to as pseudo-Meigs' syndrome.

Answer 256 (G) Dermoid cyst

An ovarian dermoid cyst "benign cystic teratoma" is a benign tumour descending from germinal cells. In most cases, dermoid cysts are unilateral, but they are bilateral in 10% to 15% of cases. Dermoid cysts can be composed of elements descending from all three of the germinal layers. Ultrasound appearances are often characteristic because of the presence of a highly reflective dermoid plug (a Rokitansky nodule), which is the solid element within the cyst that contains hair follicles, sebaceous glands, fat, and calcified or ossified elements. It usually forms an acute angle with the wall of the cyst and can produce acoustic shadowing due to the presence of hair, calcium, or bone.

Answer 257 (A) Endometrioma

An endometrioma, endometrioid cyst, endometrial cyst, or chocolate cyst is caused by endometriosis, and formed when a tiny patch of endometrial tissue (the mucous membrane that makes up the inner layer of the uterine wall) bleeds, sloughs off, becomes transplanted, and grows and enlarges inside the ovaries. Symptoms are typical for endometriosis.

Answer 258 (J) UTI

Symptoms of dysuria, haematuria and frequency are typical for UTI. PID is a differential diagnosis but no other clue would lead to PID in the question except that she is sexually active. However pyelitis is common in sexually active women.

Answer 259 (H) Tubo-ovarian abscess

Tubo-ovarian abscess (TOA) is an abscess involving the ovary and Fallopian tube. It most often arises as a consequence of pelvic inflammatory disease (PID). However, TOA can also develop following pelvic surgery, or as a complication of PID. Treatment modalities for TOA include antibiotics, guided drainage, and surgery.

Answer 260 (A) Hyperemesis gravidarum

Up to 2 in 100 of pregnant women suffer sickness and vomiting which is prolonged and very severe and causes them to become dehydrated. They often need to be admitted to hospital for intravenous fluids and other treatment. The exact cause of the sickness is not known. It is probably due to the hormone changes of pregnancy. Nausea and vomiting tend to be worse in twin and multiple pregnancies where hormone changes are more pronounced.

Answer 261 – (G) – Pregnancy induced hypertension

Pregnancy-induced hypertension (PIH) is a form of high blood pressure in pregnancy. It occurs in about 5 percent to 8 percent of all pregnancies. It is also called pre-eclampsia, most often occurring in young women with a first pregnancy. It is more common in twin pregnancies, in women with chronic hypertension, pre-existing diabetes, and in women who had PIH in a previous pregnancy.

Usually, there are three primary characteristics of this condition, including the following:

- high blood pressure (a blood pressure reading higher than 140/90 mm Hg, or a significant increase in one or both pressures)

- protein in the urine

- oedema (swelling)

Eclampsia is a severe form of pregnancy-induced hypertension, occurring in about one in 1,600 pregnancies, and develops near the end of pregnancy in most cases.

Problems occur in some pregnancies that may develop as a result of PIH such as placental abruption (premature detachment of the placenta from the uterus). PIH can also lead to foetal problems including intrauterine growth restriction (poor foetal growth) and stillbirth. If untreated, severe PIH may cause seizures and even death in the mother and foetus.

Answer 262 (E) Gastroenteritis

It is inflammation of the gastrointestinal tract, involving both the stomach and the small intestine and resulting in acute diarrhoea. The inflammation is caused most often by an infection from certain viruses or less often by bacteria, their toxins, parasites, or an adverse reaction to something in the diet or medication. Worldwide, inadequate treatment of gastroenteritis kills 5 to 8 million people per year and is a leading cause of death among infants and children under 5. At least 50% of cases of gastroenteritis due to foodborne illness are caused by norovirus. Another 20% of cases, and the majority of severe cases in children, are due to rotavirus.

Answer 263 – (D) – Hydatidiform mole

Classic clinical findings in hydatidiform moles include vaginal bleeding, anaemia, hyperemesis gravidarum, excessive uterine enlargement for the date of pregnancy, and pregnancy-induced hypertension (pre-eclampsia). Hyperthyroidism may develop secondary to a cross-reaction of beta-hCG with thyrotropin as a consequence of their shared alpha subunit.

Complete hydatidiform moles (CHMs) have a diploid chromosomal pattern, with all chromosomes being derived from the father by means of either monospermic or dispermic fertilization. In monospermic fertilization, a single haploid sperm fertilizes an ovum lacking a nucleus and then duplicates its chromosomes. Monospermic fertilization always results in a 46XX karyotype, because 46YY zygotes lack certain X-linked genes that are essential for development. In dispermic fertilization, 2 sperm fertilize an ovum lacking a nucleus. Dispermic fertilization may result in either a 46XX or a 46XY karyotype. A 46XX karyotype is found in 90% of CHMs. This finding indicates that monospermic fertilization is the dominant genetic mechanism.

Answer 264 (F) Multiple pregnancy

Multiple pregnancy occurs when two or more ova are fertilised to form dizygotic (non-identical) twins or a single fertilised egg divides to form monozygotic (identical) twins.

In dizygotic multiple pregnancies, each foetus has its own placenta (either separate or fused), amnion and chorion. In monozygotic multiple pregnancies, the situation is more complex depending on the timing of the division of the ovum.

Normal incidence of twins is 1 in 90 pregnancies (approximately 1/3 are monozygotic) and of triplets 1 in 8100 pregnancies. However, use of in vitro fertilisation (IVF) and ovulation induction techniques has greatly increased the incidence of multiple pregnancies. Figures from the North of England twins register suggest a twinning rate of 13.6–16.6/1000 maternities (or 1 in 60–74 pregnancies).

Answer 265 (K) Immediate laparotomy

The patient is haemodynamically unstable so the high probability of ectopic pregnancy will necessitate immediate laparotomy to control the bleeding and restore haemodynamic stability.

Answer 266 (A) Pelvic ultrasound

It is always important to perform pelvic ultrasound to differentiate between different types of miscarriage based on foetus viability. Ultrasound imaging, also called ultrasound scanning or sonography, involves exposing part of the body to high-frequency sound waves to produce pictures of the inside of the body. Ultrasound exams do not use ionizing radiation (as used in x-rays). Because ultrasound images are captured in real-time, they can show the structure and movement of the body's internal organs, as well as blood flowing through blood vessels.

Probably the most exciting and gratifying transvaginal ultrasound test for both the technologist and the patient is the exam for early pregnancy. This check is for the presence of an embryo, foetus and foetal heart beating. If it is a very early pregnancy (less than 5 weeks) then only a yolk sac may be noted. At about 6 weeks, a heartbeat can usually be noted and the embryo is visible unless there is missed miscarriage.

Answer 267 (L) ANTI-D administered intramuscularly

Anti D is used to prevent antibody formation after a sensitization event.

Answer 268 (D) Laparoscopy and salpingotomy

The patient has got an ectopic pregnancy. Based on her previous history laparoscopy or laparotomy is the best option. But there is no need for laparotomy as it is not mentioned that she is haemodynamically unstable.

Answer 269 (J) Transfusion with type O negative blood

Patient needs immediate resuscitation and that will entail securing an IV line and giving O negative blood.

Answer 270 (F) Endocervical swabs for culture and sensitivity

Immediate management before starting empirical treatment with antibiotics should include endocervical swabs to look for infection.

Answer 271 (G) Intra-uterine growth restriction

Betablockers are known to cause intra-uterine growth restriction, neonatal hypoglycaemia, and bradycardia; the risk is greater in severe hypertension.

Intrauterine growth restriction (IUGR) is a condition where a baby's growth slows or ceases when in it is in the uterus. It is part of a wider group – SGAs – small for gestational age foetuses – which include foetuses that have failed to achieve their growth potential and foetuses that are constitutionally small. Approximately 50%–70% of foetuses with a birthweight below tenth centile for gestational age are constitutionally small. The lower the centile for defining SGA, the greater the likelihood of IUGR. On the other hand, a foetus with growth restriction may not be SGA.

Answer 272 (I) Premature closure of foetal ductus arteriosus

With regular use of Ibuprofen closure of foetal ductus arteriosus *in utero* and possibly persistent pulmonary hypertension of the newborn can occur. Patency of the ductus arteriosus is maintained during gestation by locally produced and circulating prostaglandins. As gestation proceeds, the ductus becomes less sensitive to dilating prostaglandins and more sensitive to constricting factors such as prostaglandin synthetase inhibitors.

Foetal ductus arteriosus closure or constriction is caused by maternal medication of prostaglandin synthetase inhibitor or corticosteroid.

Answer 273 (A) Spina Bifida

Valproate can produce teratogenic effects such as neural tube defects (e.g., spina bifida).

It has the highest risk of birth defects of any of the commonly-used antiepilepsy drugs. The risk of birth defects is two to five times higher than other frequently-used anti-epileptic drugs (absolute rates of birth defects are 6–11%). Children born to mothers using valproate have significantly lower I.Q. scores (9 points). However, some epilepsy can only be controlled by valproate.

Women who intend to become pregnant should be switched to a different drug using combined therapy if possible, which takes several months. Women who are already pregnant and taking a high dose of valproate should try to lower their dose. Valproate has also been recognised as sometimes causing specific facial changes ("facial phenotype") termed "foetal valproate syndrome".

Answer 274 (D) Infant motor and mental developmental delay

There is a relationship between thyroid levels in the mother and brain development of her child. Before birth a baby is entirely dependent on the mother for thyroid hormone until the baby's own thyroid gland can start to function. This usually does not occur until about 12 weeks of gestation. Thus, hypothyroidism of the mother may play a role early on, before many women realize they are pregnant! In fact, the babies of mothers who were hypothyroid in the first part of pregnancy, then adequately treated, exhibited slower motor development than the babies of normal mothers. However, during the later part of pregnancy, hypothyroidism in the mother can also have adverse effects on the baby. These children are more likely to have intellectual impairment.

Answer 275 (E) Stress urinary incontinence

Stress incontinence is the most common form of urinary incontinence. It is estimated that about three million people in the UK are regularly incontinent. Overall this is about 4 in 100 adults, and well over half of these are due to stress incontinence. Stress incontinence becomes more common in older women and as many as 1 in 5 women over the age of 40 have some degree of stress incontinence.

Stress incontinence develops because the pelvic floor muscles are weakened. Small amounts of urine may leak, but sometimes it can be quite a lot and can cause embarrassment. Urine tends to leak most when coughing, laughing, or during exercise.

Answer 276 (F) Uterine prolapse

If the prolapse causes the cervix or the skin that lines the vagina to protrude from the vagina, this can lead to ulceration, bleeding and infection. If the prolapse affects the bladder or the urethra, complications may occur such as urine infections, incontinence of urine and retention of urine. If the prolapse affects the rectum, there can be difficulty passing stools or stool incontinence.

Answer 277 (A) Detrusor instability

Detrusor instability is characterised by uncontrolled contraction of the bladder wall (detrusor muscle) producing urgency and sometimes leakage (urge incontinence). Involuntary detrusor contractions cause urgency and urge incontinence, often with frequency and nocturia.

Answer 278 (D) Vesico-vaginal fistula

The clinical history of vesico-vaginal or ureterovaginal fistula is usually straightforward. Typically, a gynaecologic procedure, such as hysterectomy, is involved. Often, the operation is reported to have been technically challenging. Poor intra-operative exposures, coupled with heavy bleeding at the operative site, are often risk factors. Associated bladder injury may have occurred and may have been repaired.

Patients with vesico-vaginal fistula often report painless unremitting urinary incontinence. This is also called total, or continuous, incontinence. Urinary incontinence may be exacerbated during physical activities, leading some women to confuse this with stress incontinence.

Answer 279 (E) Direct maternal death

Maternal mortality is defined as death of either a pregnant woman or death of woman within 42 days of delivery, spontaneous abortion or termination, providing the death is associated with pregnancy or its treatment.

Direct deaths are defined as those related to obstetric complications during pregnancy, labour or puerperium (6 weeks), or resulting from any treatment received. The most common causes of direct deaths were thromboembolism, haemorrhage, early pregnancy/ ectopic pregnancy, pregnancy-related hypertension, sepsis, anaesthesia, and amniotic fluid embolism.

Indirect deaths are those associated with a disorder the effect of which is exacerbated by pregnancy. The most common cause of indirect deaths was cardiac illness, having overtaken psychiatric problems. Late deaths occur ≥ 42 days after end of pregnancy.

Answer 280 (C) Coincidental maternal death See explanation 279 above.

Answer 281 (J) Indirect maternal death See explanation 279 above.

Answer 282 (D) Late maternal death See explanation 279 above.

Answer 283 (B) Stillbirth

Foetal mortality refers to stillbirths or foetal death. It encompasses any death of a foetus after 24 weeks of gestation or 500 gm.

Early neonatal mortality refers to a death of a live-born baby within the first seven days of life, while late neonatal mortality covers the time after 7 days until before 28 days.

Answer 284 (G) Early neonatal death See explanation 283.

Answer 285 (N) Late neonatal death See explanation 283.

Answer 286 (N) Edward's syndrome

Trisomy 18 (T18) (also known as Trisomy E or Edward's Syndrome) is a genetic disorder caused by the presence of all or part of an extra 18th chromosome. It is the second most common autosomal trisomy, after Down's Syndrome, that carries to term.

Answer 287 (G) Gastroschiasis

Gastroschiasis means 'stomach cleft'. It is a congenital defect of the abdominal wall, usually to the right of the umbilical cord insertion. Abdominal contents herniate into the amniotic sac, usually just involving the small intestine, but sometimes also the stomach, colon and ovaries. Unlike exomphalos, there is no covering membrane. Exomphalos literally translated from the Greek means 'outside the navel'. It is also called an omphalocoele. It is a congenital abnormality in which the contents of the abdomen herniate into the umbilical cord through the umbilical ring. The viscera, which often includes the liver, is covered by a thin membrane consisting of peritoneum and amnion.

Answer 288 (E) Kleinfelter's syndrome

Those affected have an extra X chromosome (47XXY, 48XXYY polysomy or a mosaic 47XXY/46XY) and this extra chromosome material forms a dense chromatin mass in the nuclei of somatic cells – the Barr body. Advanced maternal or paternal age increases the risk for the XXY chromosome, but only slightly. Half the time the extra chromosome comes from the father. Kleinfelters' are tall (around six feet), with small testes or hypogonadism, unable to produce sperm, sparse facial and body hair and gynaecomastia.

Answer 289 (L) Congenital adrenal hyperplasia

21-hydroxylase deficiency is the cause of about 95% of cases, and is characterised by cortisol deficiency, with or without aldosterone deficiency, and androgen excess.

Clinical severity depends on the degree of 21-hydroxylase deficiency. The classic forms present in childhood with marked overproduction of glucocorticoids and adrenal androgens.

Female infants show the classic form: ambiguous genitalia with an enlarged clitoris and a common urogenital sinus in place of a separate urethra and vagina. The internal female organs are normal. Because of the ambiguous genitalia, girls with the salt-losing form of adrenal hypoplasia are usually diagnosed before they experience the salt-losing adrenal crisis in the neonatal period.

Answer 290 (K) Anencephaly

Anencephaly is a defect in the closure of the neural tube during foetal development. The neural tube is a narrow channel that folds and closes between the 3rd and 4th weeks of pregnancy to form the brain and spinal cord of the embryo. Anencephaly occurs when the "cephalic" or head end of the neural tube fails to close, resulting in the absence of a major portion of the brain, skull, and scalp. Infants with this disorder are born without a forebrain and a cerebrum. A baby born with anencephaly is usually blind, deaf, unconscious, and unable to feel pain.

Answer 291 (J) Turner syndrome

It is caused by absence of a set of genes from one short arm of one X chromosome. It can be due to absence of one X chromosome – the 45X or (X0) karyotype (about two thirds have an absent paternal X chromosome); or as a mosaic (15%), eg 45X/46,XX or 45,X/47,XXX.). Classic features are short stature (spontaneous final height is c.139–147 cm) gonadal dysgenesis (primary and secondary amenorrhoea) and lymphoedema. Newborn infants may be recognised because they have lymphoedema of hands and feet and excessive skin at nape of neck.

Answer 292 (I) Androgen insensitivity syndrome (AIS)

Androgen insensitivity syndrome (AIS), also referred to as androgen resistance syndrome, is a set of disorders of sex development caused by mutations of the gene encoding the androgen receptor. The set of resulting disorders varies according to the structure and sensitivity of the abnormal receptor. Most forms of AIS involve a variable degree of undervirilization and/or infertility in XY persons of either gender. A person with complete androgen insensitivity syndrome (CAIS) has a female external appearance despite a 46XY karyotype and undescended testes, a condition once called "testicular feminization" a phrase now considered both derogatory and inaccurate.

Answer 293 (L) Cytomegalovirus

The incidence of primary maternal CMV infection in pregnant women varies from 0.7% to 4%. Pregnant women who are infected with CMV rarely have symptoms, but rather their developing baby may be at risk for congenital CMV disease.

The average transmission rate is 40%. Of the 40% of babies who become infected, only 10% show signs of congenital CMV after primary maternal infection. The following potential problems can occur for infants who are infected from their mothers before birth: Moderate enlargement of the liver and spleen, 80–90% suffer from complications within the first few years of life including hearing loss, vision impairment, and varying degrees of mental retardation. 5–10% will present with no symptoms at birth but will develop varying degrees of hearing and mental or coordination problems.

Answer 294 (J) Treponame pallidum

Hutchinson's triad, a set of symptoms consisting of deafness, Hutchinson's teeth (centrally notched, widely-spaced peg-shaped upper central incisors), and interstitial keratitis (IK), an inflammation of the cornea which can lead to corneal scarring and potentially blindness.

Answer 295 (K) Listeria monocytogens

Listeriosis is an infection caused by listeria monocytogenes bacteria. The most common source of infection is contaminated food such as cold meats, unpasteurized milk or dairy products.

There is a risk of miscarriage, stillbirth, uterine infection, premature labour, and death in the newborn period for women infected with listeria during pregnancy. No increased risk for pregnancy loss or birth defects has been reported in women who did not have symptoms of infection. Currently, there is no evidence that listeriosis is a cause of repeat miscarriages in women. There is however a slightly increased risk for meningitis in babies, occurring 2 weeks after delivery, and is most likely related to listeria present in the mother's birth canal.

Answer 296 (F) Group B Streptococcus

These are signs of early neonatal septicaemia and Group B streptococcus (Streptococcus agalactiae) is recognised as the most frequent cause of severe early onset (less than seven days of age) infection in newborn infants.

Answer 297 (E) Varicella zoster virus

Varicella, the primary infection with herpes varicella zoster virus (VZV), in pregnancy may cause maternal mortality or serious morbidity. It may also cause foetal varicella syndrome (FVS), previously known as congenital varicella syndrome. VZV is a DNA virus of the herpes family that is highly contagious and transmitted by respiratory droplets and by direct personal contact with vesicle fluid or indirectly via fomites. Following the primary infection, the virus remains dormant in sensory nerve root ganglia but can be reactivated to cause a vesicular erythematous skin rash in a dermatomal distribution known as herpes zoster (HZ), or simply zoster or shingles.

Answer 298 (A) Human papilloma virus

Most of the time, a baby born to a woman with genital warts does not have HPV-related complications. In very rare cases, a baby born to a woman who has genital warts will develop warts in the throat. This serious condition is called respiratory papillomatosis and requires frequent laser surgery to prevent the warts from blocking the baby's breathing passages.

Answer 299 (B) A 95% confidence interval

A confidence interval gives an estimated range of values which is likely to include an unknown population parameter, the estimated range being calculated from a given set of sample data.

If independent samples are taken repeatedly from the same population, and a confidence interval calculated for each sample, then a certain percentage (confidence level) of the intervals will include the unknown population parameter. Confidence intervals are usually calculated so that this percentage is 95%, but we can produce 90%, 99%, 99.9% (or whatever) confidence intervals for the unknown parameter.

Answer 300 (G) Positive predictive value

You have the proportion of those testing positive and being identified as high risk (this will give the sensitivity and, if we knew how many had been missed, specificity). However we then know how many were truly affected, and this is the PPV – those affected in the presence of a positive test. We do not know how many were truly affected and or how many normal were falsely identified so cannot calculate the sensitivity, specificity, or NPV.